STEPPING
FROM HERRIOT'S
SHADOW

Bill Stork, DVM

LITTLE CREEK PRESS
AND BOOK DESIGN

Mineral Point, Wisconsin USA

Little Creek Press®
A Division of Kristin Mitchell Design, Inc.
5341 Sunny Ridge Road
Mineral Point, Wisconsin 53565

Book Design and Project Coordination:
Little Creek Press

First Edition
September 2016

Printed in Wisconsin, United States of America

For more information or to order books,
email: author@drbillstork.com, check out Bill's blog:
In Herriot's Shadow at www.drbillstork.com
or visit: www.littlecreekpress.com

Library of Congress Control Number: 2016950832

ISBN-10: 1-942586-16-7
ISBN-13: 978-1-942586-16-6

Dedication

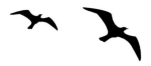

Stepping from Herriot's Shadow is dedicated to farmers and artists.

Family farmers are the foundation of our economy, and stewards of the land and livestock. They feed our bodies and are a bastion of hard work and accountability.

Painters and photographers capture the splendor as seen through their lenses to share and preserve for all time. Potters turn clay to make vessels that are beautiful, tactile, and functional. Songwriters, poets, and musicians write and perform songs to which we dance, cry, and think.

BILL STORK

Table of Contents

BILL STORK

BILL STORK

Give-'Em-Hell Harry

Disgruntled clients are an inevitable consequence of doing business. There are days when you are working for a colleague's unhappy client, and they're working for yours. There have been instances when my availability was an issue. For the last fifteen years, I've been our only large animal veterinarian. Farmers have sought services I was not able to offer, or a second opinion on an underperforming herd.

Sometimes you just don't know. It *almost* always hurts to see someone else's truck backed up to the milk house of one of your farms. But, in a few rare instances, you'd rather bathe in honey and nap on a mound of fire ants in your BVDs than pull up that drive.

Harry Schnulle was the client who fired me before I ever set boot in the barn.

Joyce Kuhl was the receptionist the day our clinic opened in 1965, four months after I was born. She was the Lake Mills Lutheran equivalent to Mother Teresa. In thirty years of service, she had been seasoned by clients and hardened by our Scottish-German founder, Dr. Robert Hance Anderson.

She slid the pocket door far enough to block the exit of the exuberant Lab. "Ah-umm, Dr. Stork, there's a guy on the phone says he's got three cows with sore feet he needs looked at this evening." Her lips pursed and eyes winced like a Little League pitcher throwing to Barry Bonds.

A plaque of the Veterinarian's Oath hangs above my desk. On graduation day, I had sworn to "use my scientific knowledge and skill for the protection of animal health and welfare, and the prevention and relief of animal suffering." It was 4:45 on a Friday evening, and I had to pick up Calvin and Paige from daycare by six. Sore feet are seldom life-threatening, and I had a hunch they hadn't just pulled up lame since lunch. I wouldn't expect Dr. Ben Graff to step away from happy hour on Friday because I turned my ankle making a post move in the Wednesday night basketball league.

Joyce was saved from the possibility of a decidedly unprofessional diatribe by the family across the exam table. I took three yoga breaths, and responded in an italicized monotone, *"Tell him I'll be there at 5:45 tomorrow morning."* I was not on the schedule for Saturday morning, but Calvin's first hockey game wasn't until 9:00. I was hoping my offer to work well outside banker's hours would buy back the cred lost by my inability to give three sore feet the urgency of a cardiac arrest.

The exam room walls are as soundproof as a voting booth, a deficiency of construction begging awareness during end of life discussions, or going heavy on the cauliflower at lunch. As Pioneer, the Roseckes' eight-week-old Lab pup, wriggled and panted, I listened for heart murmurs. Even through the stethoscope I heard, "Okay then, let us know if we can ever help you out again."

As the door shut behind Brad and Kathy, I asked Joyce the *tenor* of his response. "Well," she said, "I won't repeat every word, but there was something about you kissing his hinder..."

Counsel, enter into evidence, I *will not* do anything for a buck.

"Right before he hung up, he said if we were the last vet clinic in Wisconsin, he'd sell his cows, move to Michigan, and milk goats."

Evidently, Harry's herd gets sore feet in threes.

With fine veterinarians in Jefferson, Watertown, Waterloo, Mayville, and Fort Atkinson, it took him two years to work through the rotation. By the time I was back in the crosshairs, I suspect he'd forgotten about my first non-call to the farm.

BILL STORK

There are a few things you never forget from vet school. Professor John Foreman advised us to always back into a farm. "If you get pissed off, or the farmer chases you out the door, you look like a damn fool if you back into the manure spreader or a sixty-foot concrete silo."

Well before the backup camera, Sirius Satellite Radio, and OnStar came The Blue Mule. The 1988 Chevy WT 150 had a manual transmission, plastic seats, and roll-up windows. The cell phone was hardwired into the dash.

I swung wide at the fire number and spotted a slot in the door yard between the milk truck's tracks and the granary. I found a gate post in my rearview. The Vortec V-6 ran like grandma's Singer, but as I feathered my foot off the floor she made a throaty growl like Satchmo gargling single-malt. It was for occasions like these, and in homage to the construction worker who underwrote my education, that I cut firewood barehanded and changed my own oil. I've been known to suggest we need to give first impressions a second chance, yet I figured this was no place to waste one. I was early in the process of accumulating converts. I did not grow up on a farm, but was hoping my finesse on the clutch, the fade in my coveralls, or the callus in my palm might buy me a break.

I could have been Aesculapius, or Elvis in a Toga; it was all lost on Give-'em-Hell Harry (GHH) Schnulle.

I reached for the lever as the driver door flew open like an Alaska grizzly after a PBJ left overnight on the dashboard of a dump truck.

"Are you a (fill in your favorite expletive) cow vet?" he growled like a football coach that just lost a playoff game on a bad call.

You woulda thought we were in the Wild West looking to put together a posse. "They ain't no damn cow vets around these parts anymore." He was on a roll; there was no time to spit. Shards of Copenhagen and saliva spewed from the corners of his mouth like an Arkansas razorback boar with a tooth root abscess.

In the dairy farm dialect, the phrase, "Those vets down in 'Steubensville' are a bunch of idiots" usually translates either to "I owe them $2,500 and their office manager forbids them to set foot on this farm," or "I am more of a pain than your craziest ex-girlfriend."

With Harry Schnulle, it was option C: The United States Marine Corps. Stains in his white V-neck T-shirt suggested I was not his first victim. With a flat-top haircut and forearms like Popeye, with pressure wraps easing the onset of carpal tunnel, he was a precursor to a post on Facebook captioned, "There is no such thing as an *ex*-Marine."

I've found the most disarming approach to a raging lunatic is to respond inversely proportional to their onslaught. "Well..." I stretched, like a dog stress-yawning. Dad's words, "Shut your mouth, and let your work do the talkin'..." echoed as I formulated a response.

I thought, "I'm a professional ballerina. This isn't the recital?" But I decided it was too early for sarcasm.

"You show me the cow, if I can fix 'er, I reckon I am," I drawled in my best Central Illinois mushmouth.

Harry Schnulle remained uncharmed.

Evidently, I was supposed to jump out of the truck with bucket in hand and a hoof knife in my teeth.

"Well, grab your shit and get your ass in here 'fore the cow dies of old age."

I barely had the first patient's foot tied securely when came the machine-gun interrogation: "You go to UW? Grow up on a farm? How long you been out of school? You married? You live right in Lake Mills?"

Attention to the poor cow's foot gave me time to divide my attention and cherry-pick my response. I cleaned the manure and gravel from the heel of her inside claw, and found a black streak, suggestive of an abscess.

Should I try to break him down with sarcasm right out of the gate, or should I play it straight? I traded the left hand for a Swiss hoof knife from my leg pocket, and cleared the healthy part of her hoof.

"Naw, I'm one of those flatlanders, migrated across the Cheddar

BILL STORK

Curtain two weeks after I graduated," I deadpanned, just in case my humor-from-a-can missed.

"Well, what in the hell brought you all the way up here?" He squatted as deep as his sore knees could go, and bent until the bulging disk between L4 and L5 sent an electric fence shock down his sciatic nerve. He strained to critique what the rookie was up to.

Having isolated the devitalized area of the foot, I sunk the knife into the sole, liberating a sizzle, a hiss, and 3ccs of purulence.

"Love, initially." I paused to wipe the sweat and fetid foot juice. "But this cow is a lot easier to get along with."

As a rule, I try to fly above the "throw your mate under the manure spreader" track of barn-yard humor. In times of frustration or as an ice breaker, I'll stick my toe in. Harry jumped in feet-first with a crudely poetic analysis of the relative financial impact of boats, planes, and wives.

Had he not softened at least a bit, he'd blow an aneurism by the first visit. From the department of the obvious, he told of his service in the Marines, and that he'd served with Earl D. Woods, father of Tiger. "That man is an outright asshole," said the guy who'd fired me before he'd ever met me, and practically dismantled my driver's door on the first visit.

With his wife, Bonnie, he milked seventy fine Holsteins in a tie-stall barn. Every divider and drinking cup was solid as a soldier. The cows were bedded deep, and shit didn't hit the floor before it was scraped into the gutter and scattered with barn lime. Harry softened from the GHH I met on day one toward fuzz as our visits became more frequent.

His wife was not so warm and snuggly. I learned my first lesson on the debilitating effect of chronic pain. When we first met, Bonnie Schnulle made Harry look like Beetle Bailey. She'd beat the proverbial "bear with a sore butt" off the mountainside with a pitchfork in her right hand and a bootstrap in her left... until the day she got her knees replaced. The first time I saw her after surgery was in the clinic with their three-legged Jack Russell terrorist named Squeaks.

I initially thought Harry was foolin' around with a younger woman, and she was smiling, a first.

In short order, we settled into the realization that Dr. Stork really liked to get things done on the front end of the day, especially for farms on the periphery of the practice. Fortuitous, as Harry liked to *have* things done ten minutes before he called. The mark of a fine cow-man, there was more preventive than reactive work. Most of my calls were for sore feet, pregnancy checks, and a *little* off feed. Years in a dairy barn and the USMC had rendered a half-dozen joints bone-on-bone, but he was still plenty stout. If Harry called for a calving, you'd better eat your Wheaties *and* have a V-8.

Barns and farms can be like cable television networks. Working thirty cows and calves through the chute at the Scott Schulz farm is akin to an hour of Oprah: you'll roll away fully apprised of who's broken up, who's still together, and who is but shouldn't be. Vaccinating calves at the Larry and Betty Dahl farm is a PG-13 Norwegian RFD: you can learn all you've ever wanted to know about old guns, tractors, trucks, cold and flu treatment, prophylaxis, and chiropractic. Larry found that if he took his work boots to the bench grinder and removed the tread and rubber outside the stitching, his back didn't hurt. Each visit concludes with an Ole' and Lena joke that'd knock an iron worker off an I-beam.

Harry's place was Menard's meets Farm and Fleet. Once we'd addressed the retained placenta, displaced abomasum, or sole ulcer, Harry would regale us with home improvement tips on topics from drywall hanging, mudding, and taping, to plumbing and electrical. Before I'd stow my gear, I'd hear, "My son Chris will be taking over the herd pretty soon." Though Chris had been elusive to this point, I was certain he was a fine herdsman. That said, I'd come to treasure time with Harry and his version of "This Old House."

Harry Schnulle turned out to be one of the earliest installments of the inaccuracy of first impressions. Not only did GHH evolve into one of my favorite farm stops, he became our second call for every odd job from drywall to electrical. I was both broke and proud, but my building skills were one generation removed and supplanted by anatomy, pharmacology, and production animal medicine. I could

BILL STORK

handle matching the red, blue, and black wires when replacing a fluorescent ballast, but a shower of sparks on my feet the first time I tried a three-way switch brought an abrupt halt to my career as an electrician.

Dad always claimed, "You can't beat a man at his own trade." The Schnulle variant on Stork's postulate would be *trades*. Looking to polish up our unfinished garage, we dialed up 1-800-GHH. In the time it would have taken me to go to Menard's for supplies, he had the garage taped, mudded, and sanded. Half of which was spent bellyachin' about the crew that hung the drywall. In two coats of paint, the seams in my garage were less visible than the living room, dining room, and kitchen.

My second patient in practice was a constipated Airedale. Moose was presented by a hyper-tanned lighting rep with a trailer hitch on his Tahoe. In the nearly twenty-five years since, Gray has been the friend you could call in a heartbeat, taught my kids to water-ski, and provided every light switch and fixture in the Lake Mills Veterinary Clinic.

The reviews of Mittsy's inaugural puppy class were exemplary. Favorite part: "great material, wonderful instructor, extremely relevant." Least favorite part: "the couple with the Wyoming cattle dog (Token) were disruptive, and the basement is dark as Big John's tomb."

Thankfully, Gray had a stash of repurposed "scratch and dent" 4x4 fluorescent fixtures. In two trips to the truck, and an hour and a half, Harry had the basement glowing like Lambeau on Monday Night Football. Worthy of note: the basement ceiling is nine-inch Spancrete. Which explains why Harry brought his son TJ, who looks like he could have bored the holes and bent the conduit with his bare hands.

Like the "Free Beer Tomorrow" sign in the window of an Irish Pub, every visit Harry would assure me, "Yeah, probably next time, Chris will be takin' over." I had started to wonder if Harry had sucked too much silo gas, or was practicing some sort of existential new-age pain management: maybe if he imagined this character who would come and milk the herd, the pain in his knees and back would dissipate.

So often I had heard about Chris, my ears had gone numb. As if anything could have prepared me. We were fifteen minutes and ten cows into a herd check. I was dictating my findings on the last cow before the walkway. She had a CL on her left ovary and an excellent follicle on the right. Five ccs of Lutalyse and she'd surely be ready for love in the next three days.

Milk house doors have a rhythm and a percussion. It varies depending on direction of travel, age, construction, and whether they are closed by bungee, spring, or rope and pulley. The more mature dairyman with a milking unit in each hand will bump it twice as they scuffle through.

I heard an elbow bump and the spring stretch. Before the door whah-whumped shut, the happy rhythm of footsteps *skipping* eighth notes in the manger came closer. On task, as dictated by Harry, I backed out and waited for the next cow, paying no mind to who might be approaching.

From my periphery, I could only tell this was something I had not often seen in a dairy barn. I would double down on the task at hand, and for the love of God, I would not stare.

Indeed, Harry had not been imagining his son Chris.

As he rounded the headlocks, his skip slowed to a lilt. He extended his right hand, bent at the wrist in order to make a proper introduction; and then retracted it at the sight of the soiled sleeve on my arm. A retro-red OshKosh B'gosh bandana was rolled tightly and tied *on top* of his head. In retrospect, a perfect accent piece for equally faded summer-weight flannel. With the sleeves cut off and tied playfully in a matching bow well above his waist, his youth and farm-fitness were in full display.

Daisy Duke had nothing on Chris Schnulle.

Though devout in my heterosexuality, there was no denying the man was rockin' a shamefully short pair of cutoff American Eagle denims that were not exactly comfort cut. Scorning the utilitarian Farm and Fleet issue Tingley rubber overshoes, Chris blazed his own trail in barnyard footwear, sporting a vintage pair of mismatched high-top canvas Converse Chuck Taylor's.

Deftly switching the barn book to his right hand, he extended his left, "Good morning, I'm Chris."

I was going to need a little time to swing the vague image of the barrel-chested, tobacco spittin' mini-me I had sketched in my head... to *Chris*. Normally, palpating a cow takes fifteen seconds or less. I gripped the tail of the next cow with my left hand and raked the manure from her rectum with my right. I shook hands with her cervix and cradled her right ovary, breaking down the process I'd repeated a thousand times a week as if it were my first cow. I searched for more substance than, "Good to meet ya. Your dad's been telling me you were going to take over the herd."

I pulled out and reported that the cow was forty-two days pregnant and on her first breeding.

"Well, Harry," I stammered, "I reckon Chris and I can take it from here. You and Bonnie should get on that Goldwing in the garage and hit the road."

We wrapped up the herd check with the requisite topics of crop failure, hay conditions, weather reports, and the Green Bay Packers. I half-feigned urgency. "Well, I'd better get to the next herd check."

Koschnick Road falls off quickly to the east of the Schnulle Farm. By the time my truck appeared again, I was 200 yards out; they couldn't see me scramble for the cell phone.

Glenn Fuller is one of my best friends and the Lake Mills Veterinary Clinic staff artist. His walls are adorned with images of old men in Irish pubs at sunrise and a painting of his stunning ex-wife that will stop you cold and bring you to tears. To pay his bills, he creates things like the Klondike Bear, Nature Valley Granola Bar wrappers, and Frida.

Deeply embedded in the Chicago arts scene for the first ten years of his career and bearing a real resemblance to a young Don Johnson, Glenn knew adversity.

I was more curious than concerned. If for no other reason, fetching as it were, Chris' fashion sense was less than practical for day-in-day-out farming, and flatly uncomfortable as summer segued into fall. Glenn assured me Chris' grand entrance was every bit his signature, a mirror image of the day Harry damn near dismantled the driver's side door of my poor Chevy.

Recall, the Schnulle farm was the easternmost extension of our practice radius, and a solid thirty-minute drive from HQ. Like his father, Chris milked at four-thirty, but was even more attentive to detail. I'd try to arrive just as he hung the last unit. Cattle are creatures of habit. Like an old ladies' coffee klatch, disrupt their routine and they'll lie down in the stall and get mastitis. Make 'em a half hour late for breakfast and they'll give you ten pounds less milk, *just to show you.*

Thanks to Ms. Marilyn Claas, I found my groove early in practice. Rack-out at 4:38, yesterday's news, two bowls of cereal, and the morning constitutional by five. Marilyn paid off her farm and sold the cows a year after I arrived, but I've come to value the time. Work comes first, but if there's not a farm call or cases to research, I'll take a sunrise bike ride or rearrange the weights at the Lakers Athletic Club. To call it a workout would be somewhat of an overstatement and create an expectation of actual fitness, a state of being I've found elusive by any measure of function or appearance.

Marilyn Claas may have ensured its expression, but if any Stork's Y chromosome were to be mapped, there would be an allele that requires he be up before the cock crows. What is equally certain is that the above activities are accompanied by a sixteen-ounce Stanley Stainless vessel full of Cafe Karuba, Yuban, or on rare occasions, Starbucks Pike Place. By six-thirty a.m., I'll have 40mg of caffeine on board, effectively preventing the ascending loops of my kidneys from properly reabsorbing both sodium and potassium. If there is to be a continuous stream of thought (pun incidental), there must be a pit stop.

There are seldom organized facilities, which does not mean there is not etiquette. Discretion is accomplished on a sliding scale dependent upon urgency, the style of barn you're working in, and famil-

BILL STORK

iarity with the farmer. If in a large free-stall barn with cross alleys, you simply fall behind while the herdsman throws the headlocks for the next group. In a tie-stall or stanchion barn, you remove yourself by two to three cows and assume a forty-five-degree angle away from farmer. The T-rule of public urinals is in effect, and an audible "coffee break" proclamation is optional. A veteran will have taken notice not to set up behind the heifer with light feet and an active tail.

High school tour groups, technician interns, and farm wives invoke an entirely different set of rules. In the case of the former, you search for a location that is sufficiently remote that no part of the activity is visible to the public. In the presence of wives and milkmaids, you choose a location several paces more removed than in a single-gender barn. Without looking over your shoulder, you exaggerate the step up, in effect telegraphing your intention, and removing yourself from any responsibility as to how the lady of the barn chooses to react.

It's been twenty years from conception to completion of this particular story. Roughly 15,000 miles on a bicycle seat and a gradual rise in my PSA have rendered a tailwind more advantageous than I ever would have expected.

So, what then are the rules in a rural, yet professional setting, in the presence of a man who has been kind enough to make his preferences clear as RuPaul Charles at a feed mill?

My initial approach was to remove myself entirely, "Whoah, Chris, I put a hole through this sleeve, better run to the truck and grab another."

A plan that worked well from July into November. The advance of Wisconsin winter and its requisite dress code, the prevailing northwest wind, and the evolutionary effects of the autonomic nervous system on one's anatomy would eventually require me to move inside. The Schnulle barn was of the sixty-stanchion variety, with calf and calving pens on the west end. There was no corner to step behind. I'd try to set up at the opposite end of the barn, but Chris was young, quick, and moved with purpose.

Holding back sixteen ounces of dark roast is not to be taken lightly, yet I wanted desperately to be respectful. Recalling the Kegel exercises, I'd break stream and keep walking.

Two decades later the hurt has faded, but not once did he so much as look my way.

Poker Face

Young couples of today are less interested in traditional marriage, McMansions, and his-n-hers Lexus SUVs. It's frightening to think they have graduated, taken jobs, and co-habitated *since* I pulled my first calf in veterinary practice. They are born with tattoos and big beards, are deeply concerned about the world, the environment, and they love their pets. This generation (*not to be referred to* as Millennials) looking to adopt their first fur babies comes armed with smart phones like a third appendage. They access websites, blog posts, and Twitter streams on housetraining, proper socialization, and the most holistic, all-natural-organic-locally-sourced-gluten-GMO-grain-free-range pet food that Costco, Petco, or Blodgett's has on the shelf. By the time the litter of pups has weaned or the Paddy's Paws transport has left Houston, they've shared ultrasound images and iPhone video with everybody from Wanda in I.T. to the Helpful Hardware Man.

As veterinarians, we try to capture the energy; the first days in a new environment are crucial. We schedule the new-pet visits for at least forty minutes (three days if our behaviorist, Mittsy, is involved). We talk breed and lifestyle-dependent vaccine recommendations, parasite prevention, spay-neuter (gonadectomy) options, and nutrition. Our puppy and kitten information packages include our well-researched recommendations for groomers, boarding, and daycare services.

A nauseated dog will wait until ten minutes after we have closed to commence vomiting, and a squirrel-crazed pointer won't run into the trailer hitch on the F-150 until just before the ten o'clock news. So we include directions and telephone numbers for Veterinary Emergency Services. For the technology-averse client, or in the event Dr. Google should crash, the packet also includes a pamphlet listing normal respiratory rates and instructions on capillary refill time, in order to objectively tell medical shock from hyper-observation syndrome. If Madison the goldendoodle is feeling down and droopy, then body temperature is a crucial metric in order to tell exhausted puppy syndrome from respiratory disease. We recommend that owners designate a properly marked sacrificial rectal thermometer, *and spend the extra $7.50 to get the six-second digital model.*

I've made 911 runs to the clinic for retrievers who woke up with the midnight munchies and found everything from birth control pills to anti-depressants. In separate incidents, as the former would suggest the latter less necessary.

On a spectacular spring afternoon I was mowing and, somewhat ironically, *weeding,* at the clinic. I watched as a moderately ataxic German shepherd emerged from Tyranena Park and tacked his way through Mo's parking lot and the neighbor's vegetable garden like a Hobie Cat in a light breeze. He was followed in due time by a young couple whose ambulation was similar.

More curious than concerned, the young man remarked, "Hey, vet dude, I think somethin's wrong with our dog."

I had generated a short list of differential diagnoses, when a topless Jeep drove past, blaring the Grateful Dead. On cue, all three commenced the Kokopelli groove in the middle of the blacktop. I prescribed fish tacos, a tube of Pringles, and a nap.*

(*Actually, marijuana toxicity is a serious problem, requiring immediate medical attention if it happens to your pet. But, it's not as amusing as described in the fashion above.)

Opposite the page on Skunk Recipe (signs are awful smell and burning of the nose) is a list of common household toxins. Most folks are keen to the dangers of chocolate, non-steroidal anti-inflammatory drugs, grapes, raisins, onions, most things sugar-free, and Fox Morning News.

BILL STORK

In the wake of a recent experience I would add to the list: *diet* pills.

Benny is one of our favorite clients, his allegiance to a rival football team whose mascot bears the likeness of the former governor and a Northern European warrior notwithstanding. So deep is his misguided allegiance, there was only one possible name when he adopted a most delightful golden retriever, regardless of gender. At his eight-week exam, Fran was as cute as a calendar. Before his first birthday, Fran's boundless energy and indiscriminate appetite had earned him nearly as much notoriety as his namesake Hall of Fame quarterback.

We have tried on occasion to render our staff behaviorist speechless, efforts that have proven futile. She had advised Benny to turn his back and bring his hands to his chest in greeting Fran after a day's work, solid advice that works 99 percent of the time to discourage dogs from jumping on people. Not to be ignored, Fran would leap onto Benny's head like a sixty-pound yellow coonskin cap, and lick his nose.

As rare as a silent Mittsy, even Dr. Clark agreed this was no dog to delay his neuter.

The maple benches in our exam rooms are built by John Spaude like an Amish pole barn, wide enough for a family of four, or Benny. Most days we'd start our visit with a meaty handshake and a volley of football banter. I had withheld the reference to a "Boy Named Sue" until such a time as we'd found a strategy to keep Fran bound to the ground.

Today was different. In the face of three phone lines and a waiting room like a Haack family reunion, Claire directed traffic like Aaron Rodgers against a safety blitz. I emerged from Exam Room 2, laughing and bidding Karen Hayes and Trooper a Merry Christmas.

The holiday spirit was extinguished in a heartbeat as Claire squared up and handed me chart 3006. "We have a walk-in emergency. Benny *thinks* Fran may have gotten into something."

Her calm tone was that of a maître d at L'Etoile, but her posture spoke loudly and clearly her compassion and perceived urgency.

Benny was projectile sweating and fidgeting on the bench like Suzy Favor Hamilton. He handed Kelly a shredded wad of foil-backed packaging, "Uh, I have no idea where he found *these*; I think they're some kind of *diet* pills."

After he's greeted Benny, most days Fran moves just a bit faster than the hound dog on Hee Haw. Today his physical exam was like reading a serial number on a Tilt-a-Whirl, as he bounced around the room like Robin Williams on Red Bull. His heart was beating fast as a hummingbird, his breathing like the little engine that could, and his pupils were maximum dilated. His temperature was nearing 106F.

Without a word Kelly had started to assemble the scraps of wrapper Benny had pulled from his pocket like a slobber-soaked jigsaw puzzle.

In the moment, I was more concerned with maintaining perfusion of his kidneys, preventing a fatal cardiac arrhythmia, and seizures, than what kind of pills he had swallowed. I drew up enough sedative to slow a Missouri mule, bear-hugged him, and Megan pushed 1.5cc into his hamstring.

With the constitution of Belushi, he took several mLs of hydrogen peroxide and a half-tablet of apomorphine in his conjunctival sac to evacuate the evil. In ten minutes, a half-dozen melted grey-green capsules, the carcass of a Conrad Sentry rotisserie chicken, and the missing pieces of the wrapper puzzle formed a fetid chartreuse and orange mound on the kennel floor.

Once we were convinced his stomach was evacuated, and Fran slowed enough that I could wrap his chest and cradle his head, I presented Megan with his right front leg. She clipped, scrubbed and set a twenty-gauge catheter in a single motion. With the help of an intravenous opiate and benzodiazepine cocktail, he sank to the floor. Within seconds, the technicians were tracking his EKG, blood pressure, and oxygen perfusion.

In twenty minutes more painful than a round of golf, Kaley handed me the pink lab reports, confirming his CBC, organ panel, and electrolytes were all normal. There would be no permanent damage.

Meanwhile, Kelly had fished the scraps of paper from the pile of bile. The consummate professional, she discreetly rotated the laptop monitor. While a few pieces had made its way past the pylorus, she could clearly match the label to the image online.

As it turns out, the mysterious medication that rogue vandals had snuck into Benny's medicine cabinet while he was at work were not so much for weight loss, but more of a gender-specific performance-enhancing drug.

No, he was not hoping to *ride like Lance.*

I'm Home

Dave Mulderink had lived in Lake Mills his entire life, and recently retired from teaching physical education. I had migrated from The Land of Lincoln, and was nearing my first decade in veterinary practice. We had vaccinated, castrated, and pregnancy-checked his twenty-two Hereford cows and their calves.

For the month leading up to our herd check, Dave had a round bale feeder full of prime second crop alfalfa in the corral. In previous attempts, we had looked like poorly trained monkeys herding feral cats. Now, the cows had to walk through the chute in order to get to breakfast. They filed through like hungover college kids for chicken Kiev on Sunday morning, leaving a little time for a session of cow pasture pontification as the sun dropped to the treetops. "You know, the thing about kids these days..." We'd moved forward the exact verbiage Dave's baby boomers had spoken of my Gen X, and applied it to the Ys to follow.

Boots washed and gear stowed, I stood with one foot on the field road, the other on the floorboard. I paused to take it all in. His cattle paddock was flanked by an impenetrable overgrowth of box elder, burdock, and barbed wire to the west. Working Dave's cattle had earned me access to the mother lode: a pile of andalusite, dolomite, and quartz-flecked Wisconsin field stones flanked the field to the east. It's still the size of a school bus, after years of being raided for retaining walls, rock gardens, and stone mantles.

The sixty acres falls out of sight and returns as the neighbor's bean field, feeling more like a snapshot from Dave's Cessna than looking through the windshield of a Chevy half-ton. Just past two o'clock

BILL STORK

and a quarter mile to the east, SUVs squatting with roof racks loaded with swim floats, beach towels, and coolers full of snacks flash in the break between the Ho-Chunk Casino billboard and the Airport Road overpass. Inside, 2.2 kids are buzzing on fast food, watching movies, and kicking the driver's seat of dads who smile absently, dreaming of their first cast and an IPA.

Accounts of country vets being out pulling calves at two every morning may be somewhat historic and subject to exaggeration, or at least passively perpetuated. Cow comfort is dramatically better, farms are fewer, and farmers are more capable than ever. The updated image of on-call is that of lethargic guinea pigs, vomiting dogs, and amorous intact female cats, in addition to the fabled upside-down and backwards calves. Along with the tow-and-recovery folks, EMTs, volunteer firefighters, electricians, and every other service who sleep with one eye open, veterinarians know an unbroken night's sleep is a gift from God.

Hopefully it is also a sign that all is well.

Four years into my veterinary practice, a soft curve on County Road G and a poorly placed pile of field stone resulted in the tragic loss of Dr. Anderson, from whom I purchased the Lake Mills Veterinary Clinic. Compounded by a slumping dairy economy, my life had been dictated by the pager in my pocket seven days a week for the better part of five years.

I was humbled, fortunate, and aware that my hardship was secondary. Still, I'd find myself at Haack's, Spoke's, or the Highway A overpass by Liquor Locker, watching the constant stream of cars on I-94. The *known* of their destination or origin is… *not here*. I'd mentally stow away on the next Grand Caravan headed north. I had visions of Hayward, Cable, Minocqua, and Bayfield, but anything past Portage was no more than a mirage.

I crept past the mailbox to check for the last engineer pedaling home from Trek world headquarters in Waterloo. The truck stopped sooner than the cloud of gravel dust that sucked off the drive and through the sliding back window, adding another strata to the health papers and CD cases sliding around on the dash.

I grabbed the shifter just below the knob, and pushed it towards my hip. Before my foot let the clutch off the floor, a revelation came like looking down Lombardi Avenue and beholding Lambeau Field for the very first time.

Fifteen years ago, I had been in one of those cars, headed north on "The Highway to Heaven."

Depending on how your faith may fall, my arrival in Lake Mills can be considered the ultimate act of serendipity or predestination. Recall I was born a flatlander, bound by apron strings that had never stretched more than the forty-four miles down Interstate 72 from Decatur to Townsend II South.

I arrived at the University of Illinois in August 1983. I had just learned that Scott R. Clewis grew up the son of a tile-setter turned state senator, raised near Portage Park, in the shadows of Wrigley Field. In my haste, I was expecting Clewis Scott, having grown up in the city, closer to Comiskey, and a few shades more darkly complexioned. I still struggled to pronounce the middle name of our Sicilian suitemate from the 'burbs, Joseph Aloysius Gerbasi. And we hadn't yet hung the nickname "Worm" on our third roomie, Bill Muson.

Within my first few trips to the cafeteria, I met Barb. It could have been her sense of humor, microscopic attention span, or orange running shorts, but I was smitten.

From eighth grade on, I was the kid who was always just about to ask the girl to dance. A high school diploma, summer tan, and being relocated forty miles down Highway 72 had done little for my swagger. It took me a month to say hi at the chocolate milk cooler. By Thanksgiving, I actually sat next to her at lunch.

Her will turned out to be stronger than her legs. Bill's version of playing hard to get translated to three bushels of fifteen-dollar roses from the Chinese grocery. Even "Happy Birthday, Barbara Ann" from the campus bell tower *and* an honorary membership into the Decatur Carp Club failed to win her hand. Three years on and she had still managed to resist my charms.

We were dancing with abandon at a Thursday night Mudhens show

 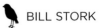 BILL STORK

at the Alley Cat bar when she shouted over Bruiser's telecaster, "My family is hanging out up by the river in La Crosse next weekend. Do you want to go?"

I didn't know La Crosse, Wisconsin, from Paris, France, but like a lab pup after a bag of hotdog bits, I said "Sure, Barb." Fourteen hours in the car and two days with her family would give me ample opportunity to chip away at her resistance.

In 1988, Google Maps and Garmin were little more than some engineer's wet dream. We'd have to rely on Rand McNally and recollection. We knew how to get from Vet Village in Tolono to Barb's house in Chicago. I asked her dad for directions.

"Oh yeah, you can go up to Sparta and bring 90 over to La Crosse, then drop down to 35," he growled, "but that'd take you way north."

"What I'd do," he continued, "I'd just bring 14 up through Coon Valley and you're there."

As far as I knew, Canada was just past Kankakee. I responded, "That's pretty much what I was figurin' on."

One thing I had learned is that city folks measure miles in minutes. "How far is it up there from your place, Joe?"

"Ah, once you get outta the traffic, it's only about four hours," he calculated.

Three hours to Chicago, four hours to the Goose Island Camp Ground.

My boss at the University of Illinois Swine Research Center was a man named Bill. Upon meeting him, your first thought was, "Now there's a man who believes in his product," followed by, "He must a fine delegator of physical labor." His policy was that I could leave work any time I wished, so long as it was eight hours after I got there. I could have feeders scraped and a load of feed started by six that morning. We were weighing Temple Grandin's "McDonald's Playland" pigs that day, but we would be done by two, easily. Eau de Swine becomes a part of you more than on you. It's not truly gone until you've molted the exposed layers. I'd take a shower and blast the big chunks off at work, then take another at home. We could be northbound on I-57 by four, and sipping a Budweiser by the fire by eleven.

If love is blind, infatuation is also deaf. To that point I had blown past more caution signs than O.J. in a Bronco, so what's another?

"If we do that, we'll just get there in time for bed," she said, which seemed logical to me. "Let's leave at midnight. We'll get there just as everyone is getting up." She phrased *her* question in the form of a statement.

"Sure, Barb!"I said as if she'd just asked me to the Sadie Hawkins. All the while I'm thinking about the prospect of 450 miles with no AC, an AM radio and seven-hour grooves, and a gallon of plastic seat sweat.

I had a fair bit of confidence that my witty banter and folksy style could win the hearts of the Hanek family. Still, I feared I could let fly with rogue "Rs" when I went to the warshroom. Such heavy affairs of the heart are best not left to fate. I picked a fifty-pound feed sack full of Illini Super Sweet, straight off the stalk, and stocked a grandma-sized cooler with twenty pounds of ice and a case of Budweiser. We would be camping but a few miles downstream from the World's Biggest Six-Pack at the G. Heileman Brewing Company, but I'd no more drink an Old Style than wear a Cubs hat. In the name of love, I may scrub the y'alls from my Central Illinois mushmouth, but I would not sell my soul.

While I do believe the key to a successful future is honesty, I had two habits that I wished to wait at least until we had the first kid on the ground to share with Barb. The first was purely physiological, and the second cultural. There is no way to emerge from working four a.m. shifts at Dave's Tackle Box *and* be a charter member of the DCC, and stay strictly within the surgeon general's guidelines. I had never touched a cigarette, but I did chew tobacco. I had committed to quitting; I just hadn't picked the occasion.

Barb's trigger to begin packing was my taillights in her picture window. I was backed up to her apartment just before the crack of midnight, just as she had prescribed. Anticipation had kept REM at bay, but I did get a bit of a nap as she scrambled to pack her swim-

BILL STORK

suit, sunscreen, and bug spray. By one a.m. we were twenty miles north of Champaign. Before the runway lights and test flights at Chanute Air Force Base in Rantoul, she was head-bobbing like a crash test dummy. By Paxton, she was lying in my lap, her soft palate snorting a chorus with every inhale.

The anticipation of the weekend would surely get me to Kankakee. With the architect of this excursion in surgical anesthesia, and nothin' but WGN News Weather and Talk to keep me awake, this was no time to go cold turkey.

To date, I'd scored a birthday kiss from Barb when I turned twenty-one. I recall oysters, strawberries, and chocolate, but I've never seen Skoal Wintergreen on Cosmo's list of aphrodisiacs. Getting caught would be the proverbial cold shower. Snoozin' and cruisin' would get us upside down in the median, spill the Budweiser and slow our progress. It might scratch the paint on the roof of the Valiant. So I'd strategically planted a tin under the visor, and left a plastic fifty-cent beer cup from CODs ovaled between the seat and the door jamb. The rhythm of reaching for the spit cup, nicotine, and a twenty-ounce Mountain Dew had me buzzed to the Chicago loop, all the way to Schaumburg.

I'd started to nod, and taken to mouthing "Amarillo by Morning" in perfect pitch along with *George Strait's Greatest Hits* cassette. Just past Richmond, Illinois, the headlights found the 12x8 "Welcome to Wisconsin, America's Dairyland" billboard.

Dad worked construction; there were no sick days or paid vacation. If he wasn't on the levers in a Bucyrus Eerie 25B setting steel, or a Cat D-8 cutting grade, there was no paycheck. At twenty-three years of age, I'd been to Disneyland and Denver. I had crossed nine state lines and still got as giddy as hearing the bell ringing on the ice-cream truck. The excitement lasted until Elkhorn, when the gauge dropped just below a quarter tank.

As Barb staggered to consciousness and squinted to find the bathroom, I walked the spittoon past the canopy lights and dumped it among the cigarette butts and Egg McMuffin wrappers. As the pump ticked off the seventeen gallons, I did push-ups and dead lifted the back bumper of the Valiant.

As I contemplated safety, Barb offered to drive. Research says: "Second only to scrotal circumference, the greatest predictor of fecundity is directional sense and stamina behind the wheel." With insecurity, modesty, and lack of familiarity, the latter seemed a more appropriate demonstration of my worth. I was bound and damn determined to pilot Grandma's grocery-getter to the shores of the Mississippi.

To this day, I struggle to consider myself a writer. I was introduced as an author for the first time in September 2015 at the Southwest Wisconsin Book Festival. It is true, in the sense that I had written a check to Little Creek Press. In exchange they agreed to bind and print my first collection of short stories. It was also at SWWBF that I learned that my genre is creative non-fiction. Within said genre we are able to take artistic license. To this point, I may have augmented reality and extrapolated the details that aren't so clear after nearly thirty years.

What is absolutely true as told, printed, framed, and stored under glass is my first vision of the great state of Wisconsin.

Less than two weeks past the summer solstice, the rising sun knifed through the ground fog boiling head-high from fields of corn and alfalfa terraced in grand curves on the south side of I-94. The leaves of the daylilies in the drainage ditches pursed to protect their pistils and stamen from the night; the corn unfurled to absorb every drop of dew. A hip-roof dairy barn and a herd of red and white cattle lay nestled in the pine valley that fell away from the highway grade. In perfect apposition, just below a Tommy Bartlett Thrill Show billboard the size of a football field, the modest steeple of St. John's Wisconsin Synod Lutheran Church kept it real.

On the north was a small barn adorned with a hand-painted mural of summer wildflowers, blue jays, and cardinals.

Summer 1988, my mission was to stick mule-kick on my slalom ski and get an attaboy from Barb's brothers, Joe and Dave. I had no more notion of living outside the 217 area code than unseating Eddie Murphy and becoming the Crown Prince of Zamunda.

BILL STORK

Proving that anything that can happen, will... In 1992, I graduated from veterinary school and took Dr. Anderson's offer of 28k, and one out of three nights on emergency. My second farm call in practice was a cow with ketosis at Joe Spoke's farm, the hip-roof dairy barn nestled in the pine valley in the shadow of the Lutheran Church.

My first vision of Wisconsin has become home.

Rambo

We were recently approached by Molly, a retired social worker who spent a career's worth of compassion in the service of people in need. Motivated to redirect her energy and exercise her love of animals, she is planning a doggie daycare and walking service here in Lake Mills.

In order to ensure that she breaks out of the not-for-profit business model, she has sought the input of potential customers and professionals. She approached Mittsy, our staff behaviorist, looking for insight and expertise. Indefatigable in her mission to ensure the proper treatment and socialization of anything that breathes, Mittsy was quick to avail herself.

I was invited to attend as well and the calendar was marked, the last Monday before Labor Day. The three of us met at Waterhouse Foods for lunch. Molly sat across the table from me and armed with pen and a virgin legal pad, her enthusiasm was infectious.

I fully expected my input would be to focus on the prevention of infectious diseases and internal parasites. We weren't quite that far when Molly commented about the dog walking service, "That shouldn't really take all that much." She was seeking input, so I pulled up my experience and that's what I gave her.

"Molly, I wouldn't start with any less than a 300,000 candle power headlamp, a fresh set of batteries, snow shoes, two handyman farm jacks capable of picking up a John Deere 4020, a snow shovel, four-foot pry bar, several sturdy sections of 4x4's, an assortment of shims, a Ziploc full of leftover New York strip, a bottle of twelve-year-old single malt Scotch, and Steve's Car and Truck Service on speed dial.

BILL STORK

She began to dutifully take notes, then slowly her head rose as she wasn't sure if I was describing watching dogs or mining for coal.

My experience as a housesitting dog walker spans two states and thirty-five years. I declared my veterinary vocation somewhere around eighth grade. Even though I wouldn't know a displaced abomasum from pemphigus for another fifteen years, from that point forward I was the de facto dog walker of Nickey Avenue. That said, three ill-fated events have served to guarantee I will forever focus on the identification of periodontal disease and exfoliate cytology.

My first patient was a geriatric cocker spaniel named Burt whose family was taking a wood-paneled Ford station wagon to the Grand Canyon. He had chronic otitis and a mouth full of abscessed teeth that he would happily attempt to sink into any shadow that resembled a human appendage, detectable through the haze of his bilateral hyper-mature cataracts. Even if those hands belonged to the one trying to snap a leash to his collar and take him for a business trip around the yard.

It's an easy extrapolation as to how he may have gone AWOL, and why capturing him was an additional challenge after we had found the wayward blind-deaf spaniel. Knowing that Burt's owner was a terminally cute seventeen-year-old dancer would only invite speculation as to why I would have contracted the job for little or nothin' and question my sincerity and devotion to my future profession.

One would think that the warm-and-fuzzy of watching Burt reuniting with his family, and the reward of a Grand Canyon keychain and T-shirt might derail the dream of vet school and launch me into a career of walking dogs. Instead, I artfully avoided any conversation that might lead up to, "We're only going to be gone for a few days, and she is such a nice dog…"

Until December 1993, when The Pope called.

With all due respect to my flatland upbringing, the minute my boots hit the ground in Jefferson County, Wisconsin, I was home. When Brett Favre took the field in relief of an injured Don Majkowski, it was time to sink roots.

Just past my elbow in the rectum of one of Joe Spoke's Guernseys, I mentioned that I was looking for a good spot to build a house. My fingertips found the pea-sized fetus in the right horn of her uterus, and I reported to Joe she was pregnant.

As we strolled three stalls west to our next cow, Joe responded, "Well, Bill, halfway down Elm Point Road, on the edge of Korth farm, there is a one-acre lot that has been for sale forever."

It was en route, so I stopped on my way back to the clinic. I could imagine a dining room picture window poised to watch the sunset over Dave's corn and beans. In the living room, I could peer over the Sunday paper and watch the deer and sandhill cranes graze Vernon Strasburg's alfalfa. Elm Point was a dead-end road with lots of weekend traffic. Winters would be quiet. Once the leaves fell, you could see the glimmer of Rock Lake from the bedroom window, three hundred feet to the north.

I stood on the crown of the blacktop in my Lacrosse overshoes with thumbs through the straps of my coveralls and brought myself back to reality. There would be impediments, not the least of which was a grove of government-issued multiflora rosebushes and a hundred volunteer box elders.

Dad summed things up. "Son, you could put on a brand new pair of Levis, and by the time you got to the back of that lot, you'd be buck-naked and bloody."

True enough, but we were no stranger to skid loaders, backhoes, chain saws, and diesel fuel. Give us two good men, a ham sandwich for each one and a Stanley thermos of coffee. With an inch or so of rain and a ten-hour day, we'd turn that jungle into a manicured lawn.

My finish carpentry skills were pretty much maxed out when I built a clubhouse around the sandbox out of old pallets and plywood in fifth grade. The University of Illinois College of Veterinary Medicine did as well as any institution could in preparing its graduates for a career in animal health. There was little gray matter remaining for business and finance. I was driving a half-ton, two-wheel-drive, Chevy work truck showing 200k on the odometer when the cable on the speedometer broke a year earlier. My Sunday go to meetin' and funeral clothes consisted of the khakis and navy blue blazer from vet school graduation, and I packed my own lunch.

Cash flowing a mortgage seemed unthinkable, but damn, that was where I wanted to push my kids on a tire swing and retire.

For my dream to become a reality was going to require The Powerball, or the Pope.

Jim Pope is impeccably dressed, meticulously coiffed and well-spoken. He may fly his plane to Mexico on Friday, race a dune buggy across the Baja on Saturday and be carving up a slalom course on Sunday; but Monday morning at four a.m., he'll be behind the desk and on the phone.

Jim was Ask Jeeves and Match.com when Bill Gates and Steve Jobs were still in a garage in Seattle. In need of a sport coat that fits just right or the best sushi in Madison? He's got a guy. Have a Saturday night and a lonely heart? Jim's got a secretary who loves animals, western swing and two-steppin'.

Find yourself staring at an acre of scrub trees and rusty rolls of barbed wire and broken bottles, the number was the same. To say Jim is a banker would be equivalent to "Jimi Hendrix played a little guitar."

His lending style has been referred to as aggressive, or at times creative. That said, have your eye on the Biltmore, and he'll hook you up for $20,000 down and 7.5 percent APR... until you're 215 years old.

Jim Pope may be a modern day Milburn Drysdale, but under the lapel of his tailored suit beats a big, kind heart. There were two things he loved more than anything: pulling his mother behind his ski boat on Sunday mornings, and his little dog Rambo on his lap, beagle ears flapping in the breeze.

What Wikipedia doesn't know is that the Vietnam veteran in the iconic 1982 film was named after an animal far more menacing than Sylvester Stallone with a knife, a machine gun, or dialogue. Rambo was an eighteen-pound Jack Russell terrorist-beagle-dachshund cross. Her black floppy ears and white tips of three toes and tail did not belie the devil within. Oh sure, she'd sniff your ear and lick your nose, but it was all a carefully calculated ploy to construct a false sense of security. Enter the room with a needle and syringe intent on vaccinating or heartworm testing, and she would draw First Blood. So much as think of a nail trimmer, and you would be unceremoniously dismantled in seconds.

All of which was lost on The Pope. Across a boardroom table in a business deal, he made Donald Trump look like a six-week-old golden retriever puppy. Bring Rambo to the vet, and he was nervous as the proverbial Dallas madam in the front pew of a Catholic church. Upon arrival, he'd be shaking like a dog trying to pass a pin-cushion. Conveniently, his pocket would ring.

With some combination of canned dog food, beach towels and sleight of hand, Rambo would be tested and protected. She'd be wagging her tail when Jim returned from icing a million-dollar deal on a condo in Tahoe while pacing a path in the black top.

The hard-wired cell phone on the dash of the old Chevy lit up as I reached to shift from third to fourth. Two Styrofoam egg cartons squeaked at the bottom of a brown bag on the passenger seat. Loaded with enough provisions to hunker-down, as last night's ten o'clock news warned of "eight to ten, with blowing and drifting."

"Hello, Mr. Bill, this is The Pope," as only he could refer to himself.

"What can I do for you, Jim?" There was only one answer to whatever was the question from the man who held your mortgage and had saved you $1500 on a well.

"I've been called out of town and need someone to watch Rambo for a few days," as if he were asking me to sweep the snow from his sidewalk.

There was a pause as I contemplated slamming the truck into a snowbank.

When the EMTs arrived, I would have neck pain and impaired speech. I had atropine on board that I could drip in one eye and dilate the pupil. Anisocoria and a case of unilateral partial paralysis would throw the neurologists off the trail long enough for Jim to find another pet sitter.

"Well, I suppose," I stammered. "When are you thinking..." as I heard a gate agent make the last call for boarding.

"Actually, Mr. Bill, I'm at the airport now," he stated the obvious. He assured me I would have no problem. She was in the basement and the sliding door on the walk-out patio was unlocked. The only thing Rambo disliked more than needles and nail trimmers was snow. (To that list we would later add 6-foot 4-inch men in rubber boots, Carhartt caps, and headlamps.) Her food was in the kitchen, he detailed.

"All you have to do is open the slider, she'll do her business and run right back in," he said.

In a 144-square-foot exam room with two skilled technicians, my chances were fifty-fifty. In a three story house, I was afraid, very afraid.

Jim had left for the airport straight from work. Rambo hadn't been out since late morning. By now the snow had started with purpose. I parked across the end of the drive to shovel and strategize. As giant flakes flew over Strasburg's corn stubble and Korth farm, they crossed the drive at a forty-five. I pushed the snow to the east of the concrete, else a drift form on the windward side.

As defeatist as it might sound, I assumed Plan A would be a bust. Regardless of The Pope's prediction – she'll just run outside and do her business – I was going to feel a lot better with Rambo securely on the end of a rope. A snap leash on her collar would be the most secure, but would risk permanent damage to one's distal appendages. A slip leash would be the most realistic.

To an eleven-year-old, eight-inch tall dachshund cross with advancing cataracts, there was no way to make my shadow look anything like that of The Pope. She met me at the sliding door gnashing and barking. So much for staying low and avoiding confrontation. I crawled through the opening and lay on the floor, but to no avail. I could have painted myself in bacon grease and held my breath until rigor mortis set in, but Rambo was going to keep at least one full room between her and me. The open floor plan of Chalet Pope made for spectacular views of sunrise, but rendered it impossible to corner Rambo in order to install a leash over her head. So much for Plan B.

Which led me to Plan C.

As I had expected while shoveling my drive, the wind had wrapped the west side of the house and deposited an impenetrable, God-given four-foot frozen dog fence just past the concrete pad.

"Rambo hates winter," says the Pope.

Sweating hard from crawling through the house in coveralls and wool socks, I pulled on my boots and hat. I gently slid the door open, and visibly retreated to the north. Rambo would know the evil was on the outside, eliminate, and run right back in the house.

Right.

At times like these, Mom would quote Robert Burns, "So much for the best laid plans of mice and men," attempting to defuse my frustration when a plan went awry.

Her cold paws hit the concrete swept bare by the wind. Standing on her hind legs, she peered over the snowdrift to know my position. The beam of my headlamp illuminated the aqua-green tapetum from the back of her eyes, and I turned quickly so as not to spook her. With one quick look to the right, she took off like Barry Sanders past a 300-pound lineman. Leaping from one boot track to the next in outright defiance of her age and athleticism, she bolted around the house, under my idling truck, out the drive and down the road.

In a flash, she disappeared into the blizzard.

Desperation and futility overtook common sense as I screamed into the squall, "Raaamboooa!" The guy who vaccinates and trims nails calls for a dog who would not come to him for fifty pounds of peanut butter-coated freeze-dried liver.

I switched to tracking mode. The snow was so deep her only option was to porpoise, or travel in tire tracks. On the high ground, the

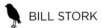

wind would drift the tracks shut in a matter of minutes, but she was scared, deceptively fast and in the lead. When Korth Highlands Road forked, she clearly took Helena Street. She continued south to where the road T'd into Elm Point Road. I ran west to Shulz's drive, then back east to the boat launch. There were no dog tracks in the tire ruts, and no sign of the little black dog, as far as the beam of my headlamp could reach. The trail had gone cold.

Fighting panic, I retraced my steps to the last confirmed track, intent on studying every inch. Just as Indian Terrace met Helena Street, there was a line of white pine that functioned as a snow fence. Past the eddy of the low hanging branches was a drift. I dropped to my knees to see a tiny set of prints scamper into the pine dander. Like a convict in a stream, I had to find her exit point.

The going was tough, and the pine trees roared an angry symphony. Between the gusts there came a decrescendo and in my heightened state of senses, I heard a shrill "Yip!" Pausing to sort reality from mirage, I carefully stepped first closer then farther in the direction of the sound, like a high-stakes game of hot and cold. Back on my knees to get closer to its origin, I found myself on the stoop of a free-standing screened porch. I wouldn't have put it past her to throw her voice like a master ventriloquist, but it seemed that I was right on top of her.

Retracing from the edge of the pine trees, there was the faintest evidence of tracks that led to the cinder block foundation of the porch. Just under the doorway there was one block half askew. Six inches: just enough to wedge a wayward dachshund. I pulled the steps and enough snow away to make room to lie on my belly and aim the headlamp.

Tragically bumping her head with every little yip was Rambo, holed up in the farthest reaches of the cavity under the vacation structure. She was far from captured, but for the moment contained. I huddled against the building and contemplated.

I cleared the snow as best I could with the side of my foot and army crawled into the opening, yet I couldn't get past my shoulders in the space. Though I chose medicine over construction, this apple didn't fall all that far. Larger buildings have been moved for lesser reasons. I surveyed the situation to find that she was indeed sealed in the space, excepting the one block. Moving with purpose, I sealed her in and promised a hasty return.

Home was only a hundred yards away. At this point, cut and paste the dog walking survival kit outlined at the beginning of this story. I threw it all on the end-gate of my truck and backed in until the tires spun. I cleared the snow from the foundation. Anticipating it would be frozen solid, I freed the deck from the blocks with a four-foot pry bar and ice scraper. Positioning a handyman farm jack under each corner, I alternated, lifting each corner 4 clicks at a time. Before there was space enough to accommodate a terrier, I would shore the hole with a shim until it was wide enough to fit a 4x4.

A small victory, in that as the patio started to rise, she would no longer hit her head as she continued to yip. So that when I went for the capture, I did not end up with a screen porch and a dozen lounge chairs on my back, I secured the situation with a bottle jack and a block on each corner.

Once again I dropped to my stomach and attempted to wriggle forward far enough to loop the leash over her beagle ears. Aron Ralston became a cult hero for amputating his own arm to free himself from the boulder and the hard place in Canyonlands, Utah. Face to face with Rambo, under a wooden deck with only my boots sticking into a blizzard, I was not thinking speaking tour and movie rights. Every few inches I would test my ability to reverse. I was four inches short when I could no longer reliably back up.

I needed just a bit more reach.

A rabies pole is an eight-foot aluminum pole with a retractable, coated cable loop at the distal end. I'd never seen one at Lake Mills Veterinary Clinic, but they have a tendency to be standard equipment in most animal hospitals and shelters, to be used when life and appendages were hanging in the balance. In this case it was hers and mine respectively... the time was nigh.

I sealed her enclosure once more, so she could not escape or go deeper; tight as Hoffa's tomb with Geraldo knocking on the door.

 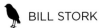 BILL STORK

County Highway S is three feet higher than Arlie Wilkie's corn stubble to the west. Jefferson County road crews meticulously keep the chicory, clover, and garlic mustard weed cut tight in the fall. Yet in some inexplicable quirk of fluid dynamics, the snow had drifted wheel-well deep from Korth's curve to Highway B.

Praying that divine intervention and momentum would suffice in the absence of four-wheel drive, I bombed down the centerline at fifty-five mph. Halfway between Shorewood Hills Road and the stop sign, there came a set of headlights. Country driving etiquette dictates in situations such as these that each driver gives the center in proportion to his machine and mission. I could already feel the snow scraping the quarter panels; my two choices were straight line or corn stubble, and Rambo was getting weaker. I chose to not speculate the commentary as I nearly brushed mirrors with a white Jeep Grand Cherokee. I watched in my rearview as it spun into the ditch.

Highway B was plowed; a temporary break so I could mentally check through the options for where a rabies pole might be stored. A hundred episodes of *Dukes of Hazzard* came in handy. I downshifted, cranked the wheel and gunned the V-6 as I flew into the parking lot, doing a 180 and pointing back at the street, increasing my chances to get back out, and looking pretty cool in the process.

There is a God, and He is there when you most need Him. On the top black shelf, in the farthest reaches, above the army-issue cotton gauze wraps, I spied a red tip and gray cable.

Throwing the pole in the middle of the Porta-Vet, I backed to the edge of the blacktop and hit the snow plow wind row across the mouth of the parking lot at twenty-five mph, praying for lack of cross traffic.

Thankful for small favors, my tracks had not yet drifted shut, and Steve's Car and Truck Service was already winching my friend Rob Larson and his white Jeep Grand Cherokee out of the ditch.

Back at the shack, on my belly under the porch, I slipped the loop around Rambo's neck and I pulled her close enough to put a chunk of New York Strip just beyond her nose. There are times to worry about pancreatitis, gastritis, vomiting, and diarrhea. And there are times to go for the capture. She relaxed just enough to come my way.

Once in my arms, she was shaking like a quarter-bed in a cheap hotel. I stuffed her under my coat with only her nose and ears protruding. I held her and she looked up at me.

I remember being enamored at Golden Gloves boxing matches as a kid. Two full-grown athletes would spend three rounds pounding one-another into submission. Before the next bout, you'd see the two combatants ringside, reliving the match and talking about wife and kids.

Rambo spent the rest of the weekend in a warm, padded, heated run. Securely behind a latched gate and fire doors.

When The Pope returned from his weekend gallivant, I had him pick up Rambo at the clinic. As she leaped into his arms, I explained the whole thing. "Jim, she just seemed lonely at home and I had some paperwork to do."

"Thanks, Mr. Bill." He handed me a bottle of single-malt Scotch worth more than my last pair of work boots.

I clutched the bottle. "No problem, Mr. Pope."

I deposited it on Rob's doorstep, on the way home.

So Molly, we wish you the very best of luck in your dog walking endeavor. As you can see, it will on occasion require more than a comfortable pair of shoes and a poop bag.

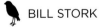 BILL STORK

A Boy Named Sue

County T north of Waterloo, Wisconsin, is straight as a runway at O'Hare. There were 2,500 fire numbers between the intersection of County I and a cow who had cast her withers. I wound the Cummins turbo-diesel up to flyin' low and punched the button on the dash to engage the Jake brake in order to save some pads and rotors upon re-entry. Not to mention, it sounds really cool.

For those who have seen the "No Engine Braking Except in Emergency" signs on the edge of small country towns looking to stay that way, and wondered, a Jake is a sort of mechanical parachute. Somewhere in the exhaust manifold, there is a gate that can be diverted to create back pressure against the pistons and slow down a big rig like a fifty-three-foot reefer with 40,000 pounds of Florida citrus bound for Woodman's, or a four-ton mobile veterinary hospital on a mission.

Next time you find yourself waiting for the sun to rise on Mulderink's Hill overlooking I-94, stop and wait. The rhythmic whoosh and whine will be broken by a deep, guttural expulsion, like big Uncle Ernie on a cheap leather couch around halftime of the Dallas Cowboys game on Thanksgiving afternoon. That would be a long-haul road warrior drifting up the exit, approaching a Kwik Trip for some Café Karuba, hot-table gourmet cheeseburgers, and a seven-minute siesta.

Sunday morning my satellite radio takes a break. The rest of the week, "Janesville, Southern Wisconsin, and Rock County's ONLY source for real country music, 99.9 WJVL" plays both Toby Keith *and* Kenny Chesney. But Sunday mornings are turned over to Big

Red, who pulls out the Ernest Tubb, Marty Robbins, Keith Whitley... and Johnny Cash.

Two miles South of Danville, and just past the big curve, we were up to the 9000s, so I backed off the throttle.

The snow was winged wide enough for an Australian road train at the driveway of N9880. A two-by-four piece of plywood mounted on a pair of "T" posts, painted green and emblazoned with a big, gold G, protected the silver rural mailbox, big as a baby's bassinet, from decimation by flying frozen slush off the Dodge County plow.

The growling Jake brake announced the cavalry had arrived. I turned down the drive past the End County Maintenance sign as Johnny lamented, "...life ain't easy for a boy named Sue," and vowed to search the honkytonks and bars until he found the dirty, mangy, dog who'd hung the moniker around his neck and left his mom.

With the truck in four-wheel high, I idled a quarter mile to the farm. The Dodge Ram barely rocked in the absence of a single bottomless pot hole, a point not to go unnoticed, as the farm drive gets pounded by everything from grain buggies hauling 450 bushels of corn and silage wagons, to manure spreaders when the cows are done with said feed. Every day of the year is a conduit for 10,000 pounds of milk a day, hauled in a 50,000-pound tanker truck. It is an active art to keep it maintained.

October rains and harvest flag the inevitable approach of winter. An offset disk or a drag pulled behind a 4020 will loosen the surface like the infield at Wrigley. A half-load of fill is feathered into potholes the size of horse tanks. On the first night the sun is to set into permafrost, the finishing touch is applied. With a box-blade on a three-point, the washboard is graded smooth, until the spring thaw turns it to mush again.

Even though the storm had not stopped until a few hours before morning milking, there wasn't a flake on the drive. Snow banks pushed two-widths onto the yard; windrows were cleaned up and piled high as a New Holland L-180 skid steer could reach around the hip-roof barn.

BILL STORK

I checked my mirrors and dropped into reverse, oblivious to the foreboding as Johnny and his dad crashed into the street, "kicking and a gouging in the blood and the mud and the beer."

The milkhouse was clean as Martha's kitchen. A John Deere calendar hung on the door turned to the current month and year. Alligator clips on all four corners kept it from curling in the humidity. In black frames hung Somatic Cell Awards from 1999, 2001, 2005 and 2006: four entire years of producing milk averaging under 100,000 SCC. Certificates of pride, evidence that you were walking onto a farm where you could walk the driveway in your wingtips and drink straight from the tank.

The plumbing that serves the twin-basin, stainless wash tanks is always a study in style and creativity. In this case, with a quarter-turn to the left on a repurposed Lucite knob from a shower stall, my dented stainless bucket was filled hot enough that the iodine steam singed my nostril hairs.

By now, you may be aware that I am prone to tangents; you may recall we have arrived at this farm to attend a cow having recently calved. In doing so she had unfortunately cast her withers, which is equivalent to tossing her calf bed, both of which are Norwegian-German dairy vernacular for a prolapsed uterus. It also means there *will* be laundry.

In the heat of restoring your patient to a more sustainable state of anatomy, there are times when a lifetime of association with construction workers* and six years on a hog farm come rushing back. You run through every illicit descriptor in your vocabulary and invent some new ones on the fly, all the while grunting like a Sumo wrestler in the throes of a prostate biopsy.

Medically speaking, the process of gestation and parturition stretches everything from the ovarian pedicle to the broad ligament that anchors the uterus itself, like a guide wire on a power pole. Mothers in the reading audience are thinking… duhh! The simple and repeatable fact that – across species – the female's external genitalia can accept the male in such a fashion as to promote procreation, then in nine months' time allow passage of offspring, and in a few short weeks be ready for another round is undeniable proof there is a superior being.

However, when things go bad, it can be catastrophic. On an occasion when a cow generates intra-abdominal pressure that exceeds her ability to retain her parts, it all falls out behind. The void is filled on the next grunt by multiple loops of intestine. From that point, it takes effort to restore order.

Imagine that Shaquille O'Neal had a pair of rain pants. Tie them at the ankle with a piece of baler twine and fill them with pork chitterlings. Hang them about chest high, and grease them up with olive oil. Now, try to stuff them backwards through a mail slot.

And so I confidently strode onto Elmer Gerstner's farm.

Over the years, I had developed a nearly bullet-proof wardrobe scheme for a job that would turn Mike Rowe's stomach. I pull my Helly Hansen, 100 percent waterproof, rubber rain pants and jacket tight at the neck and over my boots, like a farm-ready, cold weather dive suit.

In the bucket of iodine water were two bottles of calcium and dextrose, twenty cc of banamine to help her inevitable discomfort (think IV Advil), four cc of lidocaine for an epidural, and two feet of umbilical tape (medical shoestring) on an S-curved needle big enough to drive any reasonable woman to a life of chastity. Over my right shoulder was a ten-foot bull halter to anchor her front so I could work on her back end. In my left hand were five gallons of water for cleaning things up. I had two cups of sugar in a Ziploc in my hip pocket.

The Holstein dairy cow may be the mother breed of the human race, but I have yet to meet one that is house-trained. After they spend the night in the adjacent free-stall barn for comfort and lounging, Elmer brings them in for feed and milking. As they saunter, they eliminate, often mid-stride. On average, a cow eats fifty pounds of feed and drinks thirty gallons of water per day. Most of what goes in must come back out.

In Elmer's barn, there's precious little evidence.

The driveway is scraped clean and lime is spread before the first udder is prepped for milking. The gutters behind the cow are bedded deeply with fresh yellow straw.

There's something that always squared me up about a dairyman in uniform. Gerstner's was a family farm with a capital F, complete with I-bolts in the beam to hang a swing for the grandkids, and a Jersey heifer in a pen for the Little Britches class at the county fair.

Elmer was in the middle of the row by the time I arrived. I sat my bucket on the drive to exchange a handshake, the likes of which you will not find at a law school class reunion. His striped shirt was tucked into gray khakis and bound by a black leather belt. A white oval patch that read "Elmer" in blue cursive letters over his left pocket ensured you were dealing with the guy who wrote the checks.

"She's in the lean-to on the south side of the barn. Be there as soon as I pull these units." He pointed through the sliding doors.

I picked up and walked past fifty cows, clean tails, and round udders. Working conditions require the country vet to wear tall rubber boots. To ensure they can be pulled over your Red Wings, there is always a bit of slop. This was a farm where you pick up your heels so the man knows you're there to work.

I hiked the halter back up to my neck as I slid the door at the end of the barn, and pulled it closed again.

It is not until times like these that you start to realize all the observations that serve to size up the extent to which your existence is in danger.

There was a fifty-foot lot between the barn and the maternity pen. The snowfall and run-off from the barn roof made for a boot-suckin' mess. At a right angle from the barn was the remnant of a cinder-block wall, just high enough for a cow to easily step over. Surrounding the barn was a three-wire high-tension electric fence. Holsteins raised by hand are prone to gravitate around feed and comfort; Elmer Gerstner was not about to take chances on a jail-break.

I walked on the only firm ground, which was under the overhang, and sat my bucket down. Sliding open a hanging door that kept the prevailing northwest wind off the new mothers, I was met with a five-foot high, sturdy green gate.

At this time it is important to clarify: the *second* rule of farms and ranches is to leave every gate exactly as you find it.

Rule 1: Save thy biscuit.

Every observation I had made to this point put my risk of bodily harm squarely between zero and none. Still, for reasons I have yet to explain, as I stepped into the pen, I pulled the hanging door just far enough onto its bracket to keep the wind from sucking it like a sail and pulling it off its tracks.

And, in flagrant violation of Rule Number 2, I draped the chain over the gate, without latching it.

My patient faced away from me, licking her calf. The handle clanked onto the rim of the stainless-steel bucket. Like a wrestler hearing the bell, she spun so fast the centrifugal force of her uterus nearly knocked her from her feet.

Clearly confusing the guy there to fix the problem for the one who caused it, she gathered in an instant and charged.

She buried her head in my solar plexus and drove me through the gate I had not latched, and the door I had failed to hook.

In retrospect I'm amazed at the sheer volume of thoughts that can cross a person's mind in a relatively short, and otherwise perilous, period of time.

Feeling like Dick the Bruiser riding André the Giant's shoulder across the ring headed for the turnbuckle, I contemplated my options: it would be important not to let her body-slam my lumbo-sacrum across the old block wall. Sore knees have robbed my ability to squat in front of a cow; paralysis would be even more of an impediment.

Johnny's dad kicked like a mule and bit like a crocodile...

If she deposited me in the mud, there would surely be blood, and a beer would eventually go down nicely.

BILL STORK

The problem was that a dismount in the slop would negate my legendary footwork in trying to escape. Not wanting to be responsible for the escape of an otherwise prized cow, I took comfort in the earlier observation that the far pasture gate was closed. I clung to the five gallons of water. Clearly after being charged by a 1400 pound cow, the last thing you want to do is have to walk all the way back to the milkhouse and refill.

I've been to a rodeo or two, and the cowboy's ultimate goal is the proverbial eight-second ride. They're clinging to the back of an intact male Brahman, not the head of a recently calved Holstein. But in my defense, they have a rope, firm footing and a couple clowns for protection.

As unlikely as this scenario seemed, it would be better if it were witnessed. I wasn't necessarily thinking bail out, but it might be cool for Elmer to see how this all went down.

It seemed like an hour from the time I heard the barn door roll open and saw Elmer in my peripheral vision. He stuck out his chest, waved his arms and growled, "Damn it Bridgette. Doc is here to help you."

With that, she shrunk and sulked like a scolded kindergartner, and I slid off her head without so much as a scuff.

Walter Peyton always prided himself in getting up before the 250 pound linebacker who had tackled him.

Neurologically intact and unbroken, I asked Elmer, "What do you think the Packers' chances are against the Bears at Lambeau tonight?"

"Depends on *which* Favre shows up," Elmer grinned.

While circling the lot high-centered on the crown of Bridgette's head and clinging to her ears, I'd had a fully developed thought about balance, in the cosmic sense. Replacing a cow's uterus under ideal conditions can be a Herculean physical task. Given the headwinds on the front end of this little obstetrical catastrophe, surely the gods would smile. And they did. Though the displacement was complete, it was also clean.

"What do you think, run her into her stanchion in the barn?" Elmer asked.

Having had so much success to this point, "Sure," I replied.

We did just that and she was the model patient. The calcium in her vein induced contraction of the uterus and the sugar caused it to sweat and shrink. We scrubbed it clean, and with a few grunts perfectly apropos for a Sunday morning, textbook anatomy was restored.

Credit when it is due. At or near seventy years of age, the construction worker to whom I owe most of my ethic and education made the executive decision that cursing was crude. No patches, no hypnosis, just cold turkey. In one swoop, he scrubbed his language. I aspire to that policy, but have yet to adopt it as a whole.

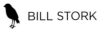

When in Roam...

Find yourself wedged under a brush hog that successfully located the long-lost sewer cover, overgrown by burdock and thistle, and Gary Edmonds is the friend who will lay an 11/16th box end in your palm and be on the top side with a socket to wrestle the mangled blade off.

Google Maps says it's 180 miles and three hours from his door to mine. If I called and said, "I need..." he'd drop his fork and phone and head north. He and his wife Dianne would be pulling down my drive in two and a half hours.

Gary grew up smack between the Illinois and Mississippi Rivers in Pittsfield, Illinois, one hundred miles east of my hometown of Decatur. He is the epitome of a family man: a husband to his wife, a coach and father to his daughters, and a brother to his siblings as well as his friends. So much so, that in order to preserve his carcass and provide for his family, he has traded his Wranglers, ropers, and one-ton dually for a Toyota, khakis, and a laptop. The man who is far more comfortable on a tractor or a roof with a nail gun is now an Insurance Man.

The thread he will staunchly maintain to his porcine past is an outright, yet elegant, refusal to eat so much as a bite of chicken. Under any circumstances.

While not physically imposing, Gary walks with purpose and speaks decisively with a nearly concert baritone. Like many, the years and life behind a desk have served to round his shoulders and soften his hands. The inevitable march of time has thinned and peppered the hair on his head, but the physical feature the caricature artist at Disney would draw first, is his mustache. The full-on horseshoe variety covers his upper lip and extends past his chin, later emulated and made popular by Hulk Hogan. I have no evidence he wasn't born with it. He stood out like an electrical engineer in a Georgia Baptist choir in his eighth grade yearbook.

Gary and I met in 1986 at the University of Illinois Swine Research Center (SRC). SRC was a 500 sow farrow-to-finish research laboratory, one of three hog farms, a horse, sheep, dairy, and beef operation that were known collectively as South Farms.

SRC sits just past Assembly Hall, where the mighty "Flyin' Illini" came within a game of a NCAA championship in 1989, and a soft southern breeze past Memorial Stadium, where Ray Nitschke and Dick Butkus once struck fear and crushed bones. (Chancellor Phyllis Wise recently appointed an independent commission to study why high-value academic and athletic recruits from the Chicago public and parochial school system are hesitant to commit to the University of Illinois.)

At SRC scientists conducted research on feed efficiency, carcass quality, and genetics. We compared weight gain and feed efficiency of groups of pigs raised in simple environments and darkness to those in stadium lights and Dale-designed porcine playgrounds. We were early to the party in the field of Environmental Physiology, seeking to design animal containment facilities that maximized animal comfort, under the tutelage of a professor named Stanley Curtis.

Dr. Curtis furthered a very simple concept that largely defines animal agriculture to this day, called the Welfare Plateau. Simply put, the kinder we are to animals, the more healthy and productive they will be. Dr. Curtis was an amazing man, known for having an enormous backside, a photographic memory, and a graduate student named Temple Grandin. His hinder was a fortunate anatomic adaptation, as he was never without an entourage of academics in his wake, and prone to sudden stops.

In her early days, Temple researched the effects of running pigs into a chute and squeezing them – a technique she eventually showed to have a significant calming effect on dozens of species. Since that time, she has gone on to be the world's leading authority on the humane handling of production animals, and has written several books on companion animal behavior. Temple is a heroine to families worldwide: she was born autistic, and is one of the first to describe the condition from the inside out. It can be said, without a thread of exaggeration, that she has done more to further the future of children with autism than anyone before her or since.

SRC was run by a man named Bill. At least, in the sense that he had the front office, two filing cabinets and a phone. His Oklahoma drawl and physique spoke of a man who believed in his product. "Boss Man" was amiable as the day was long. However, when it came to running a farm, he couldn't find his butt with both hands.

Fortunately, SRC was staffed by a full-time cast of characters who were as diverse as they were capable. Dale was the maintenance man and metal-fabricating magician. There are rumors that he blames me to this day for any missing tools (I drew my last paycheck in 1990).

Diane ran the farrowing barn and nursery. She only took days off to make emergency trips to Memphis, as her brother Leroy/Elvis/Bubba had multiple personality disorder and a penchant for hostile takeovers of Graceland during his weeks as The King.

Scotty ran the breeding barn, built his own home, got married and had kids in diapers, grade school and middle school by an age when most of us are getting the hang of shaving.

So in the University of Illinois hog farm hierarchy, you have Oklahoma Bill and the professors at the top, the graduate students and full-time farm crew in the middle, and Gary and I bringing up the rear, technically classified as grunts. This classification was confirmed by the sizzle of a three-foot cattle prod vaporizing the sweat between my clavicles a fraction of a second before I grunted like being tackled by Clay Mathews and hit the woven wire deck of the trailer. I figured it was either some sort of rite of passage or payback for a quip that questioned the preferences of Dale forty-eight hours into my tenure at SRC.

Gary and I were deeply concerned with the ultimate goal of putting the chops and brats on your Weber, as humanely and efficiently as possible... and water skiing.

In order to appreciate the vitality of our roles in the execution of the world-class research taking place at SRC, you'll need a brief lesson in porcine behavior, anatomy, and nutrition as it relates to agricultural engineering.

Two of the most important measures of porcine production are weight gain and feed efficiency. Scientists are charged with the responsibility of weighing what goes into the pig, and measuring how quickly and lean they grow. Kind of a scientific version of pencil marks on the basement door frame on the first day of school, if mom were to count every bowl of Cheerios and chocolate chip cookie in between.

Mark Twain said, "Never teach a pig to sing; it wastes your time and annoys the pig." Mittsy Voiles, CPDT-KA (she's really smart and knows about these things), said they are cute, funny, and smarter than dogs.

Chefs will debate the best way to prepare a pig; peach demi-glace and Riesling vs. Arthur Bryant's barbecue and an IPA.

What has never been suggested is they are delicate, neat, or polite. Gary Edmonds and Willy Stork will testify.

Agricultural engineers have worked for years to design a feeder that will deliver grain to a pen of pigs uniformly without being destroyed. In decades, the design has changed little. Feed is poured in the top, regulated by a baffle at the bottom, and covered by a lid.

As alluded to by Mittsy, pigs are smart enough to lift the lid if you installed a touch pad and six-digit entry code. The association they have yet to make is what happens when they mangle the lid or get it stuck in the up position. First, there will be mayhem as the lid is open for free access. Then things get ugly.

Given the proper pen and spacing, pigs are relatively good at not soiling the area where they lay and eat. There are exceptions.

Best-selling author and part time pig farmer Mike Perry advises to limit your time behind a sneezing cow. Similarly, never place your breakfast behind a gilt (young female pig). If the urge strikes at the exact moment that a penmate is breakfasting in front of a failed or mangled feeder lid, she's going to get "piss in her cornflakes."

That is the time when the grunts become a gilt's best friend.

Dedicated and skilled as they were, the full-time staff at SRC are state employees. As such, they tended to stick to the hours of 8:00 to 4:00 and the time clock on "Boss Man's" desk. Especially on appointed water ski days, Gary and I would be "all hands on deck" by five a.m. Armed with the second half of a forty-eight ounce Mountain Dew Mega-Buddy from 7-Eleven, we would descend on the grower and finisher barns.

Dale had fabricated high-tech feeder rods. Exquisite in their design, they were a three-foot piece of steel with hand loop on one end and flattened hook at its terminus. Yet there is only one tool that could efficiently dig feed, manure, and urine from the bowls: your hand. Preferably the hand opposite the one you used to install the first dip of Skoal.

Off the clock, Gary and I talked for hours about girls, water skiing, music, and girls. On the University's dime, we were all business. Though it was never spoken, we were bound and damn determined that when the first of the full-time farm crew kicked up the gravel dust, every pig was eatin' clean. Research could commence at the top of the clock. The integrity of the work at SRC and the welfare of the herd was our first motivation; getting to the lake, just a perk. Having arrived three hours early, Gary and I could be on Lake Decatur by the time the full-timers hit the shower, on the end of a sixty-five foot tow rope, kicking up a massive wall of muddy water.

As glamorous as our position was not, there were jobs we jockeyed for: mowing grass, trimming weeds, spreading gravel in the parking lot potholes, and moving irrigation pipe. To get a sense of what we were up to with the irrigation pipe, imagine you had a lawn sprinkler with a dozen heads, served by a four-inch pipe. Instead of city water from the hydrant, you were pumping from the manure pit with a hundred-horse John Deere. One day Gary and I failed to calculate the velocity of a Northwest breeze *and* placed the pipeline 50 feet from 4th Street. The rather hostile gestures from the profs in their Mercedes as they frantically rolled up their windows rendered Boss Man's desk phone a rather busy unit, the minute they hit the office.

You may sense a trend. Outdoor jobs were a premium, though the air was only "fresh", by comparison to the barn.

There was no job more desirable than hauling pigs from the finishing barn to the final phase of the research project. Competition among the crew was directly proportionate to the weather for the day: the warmer and sunnier, the more intense. The Meat Science Lab was on the corner of campus. Though not the most direct route, you could catch a public park, three sororities and the Intramural Physical Education Building along the way. IMPE had an Olympic-sized swimming pool surrounded by a deck the size of a football field. Chances were good, especially during summer session, you were going to see things far more attractive than a thousand pigs or Dale.

Transport was a 7x16 pigpen on wheels, drawn by a 1969 Case 530. Like a mini-van chair lift, it raised from flat on the ground to chest high. For that function, we would soon become eternally grateful. Arranged orderly – ham to shoulder to bacon – it would haul eighteen 250 lb. passengers. On this fateful day we had twenty-one. Rather than take two trips, everybody sucked it in.

I looked both ways and pulled onto South 1st Street. Grinding and skipping from second to road gear, I dropped the clutch and throttled up. The old tractor lugged a puff of black smoke, and by the time I passed the first of our unfortunate neighbors, the tires were whining against the blacktop.

My barber, an eighty-year-old WWII veteran named Wes Gillespie, called me "Duroc." I sported a full head of dark red hair, expertly trimmed by Wes – flat on top, tight on the sides. In order to keep the sweat out of my sight, I sported a blue OshKosh B'gosh do-rag, formed to my head in homage to my guitar totin' buddy, Bruiser. Caked with feed dust and manure, my favorite pair of holiest Levis would have stood in a corner without me in them. My left foot in brown rubber boots tapped the beat of "Pain as Big as Texas" on the gangway as I rolled down the road and sang out in full voice

BILL STORK

behind the growl of the tractor. T-shirt cropped cool like Kenny Chesney, I was quite the sight.

Cars passed as I waved and spit between the tire and fender, nothing could break my rhythm. The closer I got to town, the friendlier, if not exuberant, folks became. Every person I passed waved. I pulled into town contemplating how I might lure one of the bathing beauties from her Walkman and blanket to my tractor, which was not in the least bit sexy. Before I could work out those details, the afternoon took a turn.

As the first university buildings came into view, I downshifted and throttled. Northbound was a young man with his left arm and whole head out the door of his Chevy, waving frantically and pointing.

Curious, I turned to see the tender-foot bottom of the hog hauler with only fragrant evidence there had ever been a pig inside. Their exodus was manifest by the endgate swinging freely into oncoming traffic.

Immediately I thought: Will this hurt my chances with the girls? How will I get the pigs back on? What's Oklahoma Bill going to say? Other musings would follow.

Were it not for good fortune, the nature of pigs and the Ogallala Aquifer, the feral pig population of central Illinois may have started with a cotter pin placed backwards.

On the east side of South 1st Street, there was a Mazda RX-7, Nissan Z-something and a Corvette, parked bumper to bumper. I backed the trailer so the gate matched the bumper of the Mazda, and the row of performance sports cars became my crowd gate.

As for the pigs...

Beginning with the Romans, centuries before chisel plows, there were hungry people, and pigs. Where ground was too hard, dry, and rocky to pierce with a pick or a shovel, they would turn herds of pigs. In search of insects and mud, pigs instantly bury their snouts and root.

Mid-summer '88, we were squarely in the middle of fifteen consecutive 100-degree highs, and dust bowl dry. The one notable exception was the manicured and landscaped quarter-acre lawn of the University of Illinois Credit Union. Thanks to an abundant underground water supply, employees could gaze at a veritable oasis in the middle of an historic drought.

Having spent the first six months of their lives under roof and on concrete, the pigs moved with efficiency, purpose, and power. There were water lines, wires, and divots to be rooted up, as if a farsighted Paul Bunyan golfed with Babe as his caddy. The polarized glass of the U of I Credit Union reflected the morning sun and left us to forever wonder what the staff thought of a redneck in a bandana herding pigs on their lawn.

The gentleman who had waved me down had farm-smarts and two brooms. Thankfully, the nature of pigs is to move to what is familiar. Shortly, we had them rounded up and secured.

Cell phones were a decade in the future, which mattered not. I would have tried anything short of issuing an SOS back to SRC. I had no fear of discipline; it was the ribbin' from the fellas I'd avoid at any cost.

I'm pretty certain the guy who put the cotter pin in backwards is also the one frequently implicated around here when tools go missing.

BID (every 12 hours)

[Disclaimer: Some names in this story have been changed to protect the innocent. Some details have been made up entirely for entertainment. That said, the ending is entirely true.]

Dawn Francois: the sound of her *name* as spoken by Pepe Le Pew or a high school French student would conjure up images of sipping tea, nibbling croissants, and watching the sun rise over the River Seine in Paris.

The sound of Dawn's *voice* at eight in the morning conjures images of a family feud between *Duck Dynasty* and *Swamp People*, and requires Claire to bump her chest in order to keep the Kwik Trip ham-egg-cheese breakfast bagel on the south side of her esophagus, while retrieving morning messages.

Let the record show that the overfed Boston terriers of America have never known a better friend. The doctors and technicians at Lake Mills Veterinary Clinic have seldom been more entertained than when Dawn's entourage rolls into town.

November through March in Wisconsin can take a toll on your soul. Spring is the rebirth that we all live for. For some, it is the organic smell of fresh-plowed ground or rounding the north end of Rock Lake to the motion of waves, the first day of ice-out. For doctors and staff at the Lake Mills Veterinary Clinic, spring is signaled by a fleet of Toyota pickup trucks labeled Francois Paving with decals down the side and No'th Ca'olina license plates on the bumper.

Dawn and her husband Burt run a blacktop business. In winter, they retreat to their native North Carolina. At the first sight of green grass in the Badger State, they descend upon Wisconsin, spreading fliers and knocking on doors.

Brachycephalic Breed Syndrome is a group of conditions used to describe dogs with elongated soft palates, stenotic nares, everted laryngeal sacules and a poorly formed trachea. These are the dogs that look like their brakes failed at full speed en route to a brick wall. An eight-week-old, five-pound bulldog pup scrambling for treats on the exam room floor sounds like a pen of feeder pigs fighting over a bag of day-old donuts. What they lack in longevity and athleticism, however, they double in charm. Boxers, Boston terriers and pugs are universally engaging. With Dawn on the other end of the leash, they're a comedy team on par with Edgar Bergen and Charlie McCarthy. Adjusted for demographics: more like Jeff Dunham and Walter.

We generally see the boxers, Bella and Tyson, for vaccines and spring blood testing. Bones and Betsy, the Boston terriers, require frequent pedicures, and a lot of smoke breaks. Not for the dogs, of course; Dawn's aversion to needles and discomfort on the part of her dogs is coincident and in direct proportion to her need for nicotine. Grab a swab or a syringe, and Dawn will put the back of her hand on her forehead and close her eyes. Before actually fainting, she'll reach for her bedazzled iPhone, a pack of Marlboros, and a flame-throwing Bic, and make tracks for the porch.

Her five-year-old pugs, Buster and Lilly, are littermates. Buster was born with a condition called dry eye. We call it keratoconjunctivitis sicca. It sounds more medical, is nearly as fun to say as phenylpropanolamine, and totally befuddles spell-check.

Miss Lilly is as charming as her name but her ears are as narrow as her trachea.

Whether you are a veterinarian, auto technician, or a plumber, if you've got a lick of integrity you look to assess, diagnose, and cure. See the problem, fix the problem. Miss Lilly's ears simply defied our mantra.

In the process of learning how to most efficiently and least invasively manage Lilly's ears, we damn near killed Dawn.

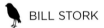 BILL STORK

We had treated Lilly fourteen days prior. If the outcome is in doubt, or the condition chronic, the best medicine is to follow up with our patients. When a tough case is turning our way, we've been known to hug, high-five or fist bump a client. If poorly, we gnash our teeth, stick a swab in something and retreat to the office to look up plan B.

As Miss Lilly approached, I observed without saying a word. (Mittsy and Megan have learned to compensate for Dr. Stork in thought.) She had no more head tilt and never stopped to shake her head. The smell of freshly baked bread that signaled the yeast infection two weeks ago was absent. A cotton-tipped swab returned from the bottom of her vertical canal came back spotless, and on deep otoscopic exam, there was not a lesion to be found.

When I looked to Dawn to report the good news I thought she would expire right on the floor.

"Thank Gawd, Dr. Stork, I ain't had a night's sleep in two weeks," she stammered.

In twenty-three years of practice, I've seen the depth of a person's love for their animals demonstrated on a daily basis. Lilly's ear infection was real, but at no time did we fear that she wouldn't come through it alive.

I must have seemed a bit puzzled.

Dawn's look was that of disgust. "Dr. Stork, your label clearly read: 'APPLY 6 DROPS TO EACH EAR, EVERY 12 HOURS, UNTIL OTHERWISE DIRECTED'."

Her initial appointment was at 3:15 p.m., when we had applied the first dose of medication for her.

5-TON

(a kinship with Fred J. Eaglesmith)

Note from the author:

Robb Grindstaff is an editor with skill and experience. He works really hard to keep me between the lines. Red boxes in the margin of the document mean I need to clean things up in order to not leave the reader lost by the side of the road. His comments are as follows for the story you're about to read:

"This story really winds around all over the place without a clear narrative arc (beginning, middle, and end) that tie together, although eventually it does come back to Fred. But it starts talking about Kenny Chesney and country music, then to Fred, then to construction, and trucks and Porta-Vet, and a long construction scene that I couldn't follow, then a cross-country trip to pick up Paige from school. Really had trouble following this one."

I replied, "Robb, I couldn't agree more, but Fred liked it."

Kenny Chesney writes about sun, sand, no shoes, no shirts, and no problems. Mr. Chesney has six Academy of Country Music awards, including Entertainer of the Year from 2005-2008. He has a collection of six CMA (Cross Marketing Association) awards. Mr. Chesney travels by private jet. A convoy of Kenworths transports a small army of technicians, stage hands, and construction workers who assemble his road production in football stadiums from Green Bay to Dallas. His *No Shoes Nation* is to millennials in ball caps what Buffett's Parrotheads are to boomers in grass skirts. They party for hours before Mr. Chesney takes the stage. His concerts are unbridled barefoot, boat drink, and bikini perpetual weekend affairs.

 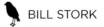 BILL STORK

A self-made star and son of a school teacher and beautician, he can always be found in the cheap seats during sound check. All-the-better to appreciate and play to the hard working folks who pay his salary.

Fred J. Eaglesmith writes:

Well he stops his horse, to get a light
and the water pours out of his hat.
He's been out in the rain most of the night
and ought to be getting back.
He's been thinking about the colour of
her hair and the touch of her hand.
And the way she quietly smiles whenever
she looks at him.

But he only gets into town twice a month
and he gets out as fast as he can.
He don't have a phone so he can't call
her up and he never knows where she is.
She smells like flowers and perfume
and tobacco and gin.
He's been in love a couple of times
before, but never quite like this.
He's been in love a couple of times
before, but never quite like this.

Fred and his Traveling Steam Show play small bars, listening rooms, and theaters from Texas to Canada, and all over Europe. They have recently upgraded to a 1990 Bluebird Motor Coach. It's been gutted and retrofitted with pumps and filters to run on waste fryer oil by the chief mechanic, bus driver, and songwriter Fred J. Eaglesmith. They do not tour in support of albums; the road is where they live.

He is known to pull 4-8 hour shifts behind the wheel and play impromptu four-song concerts for fans who recognize his rig in the Walmart parking lots where they rest. Multi-day "Fred Fests" feature concerts by singers and writers by night and a winner-take-all band-vs-fans street hockey tournament by day.

En route to a show 250k west of Calgary, the Bluebird ground to a hopeless halt. Matt and Kori panicked. No well-prepared Canadian farm boy would leave home without a spare; Fred changed the transmission on the shoulder. Grease wedged under fingernails and knuckles skinned, the show must go on.

A student of Buddhism, philosopher, painter, and poet, Fred has been celebrated, decorated, studied and honored in three tribute albums and numerous college courses. He builds towering tangible images, only to apply them to gut-wrenching metaphor. His songs have been covered by Toby Keith, Miranda Lambert, Alan Jackson, and The Cowboy Junkies. In many cases, the covers are note-for-note and every inflection intact. At open mics in coffee shops and microbreweries, he has been imitated by folk and alternative artists too numerous to conceive.

In the fall of 2012, recording industry executives offered to fly him to Nashville. They would put him up in the Vanderbilt and honor his contributions at the Mother Church of Country Music, the Ryman Auditorium. He was flattered but declined. *It fell on the same date as a sold out bar gig in Duluth Minnesota… for 85 Fredheads.*

"That was the excuse I gave 'em," Fred told a sparse but loyal crowd at the High Noon Saloon in Madison. "Those damn punk kids checkin' their Facebook status and snappin' selfies don't get my music anyway," in his road-weathered growl, always cordial to a fault.

Fred was born on a dairy farm in Southern Ontario, Canada. He tells stories of balin' hay and farming with two tractors and one battery. It was clear that eighty acres and two dozen cows could not support nine kids and two parents. At age sixteen, Fred hopped a train, bought a guitar and commenced writing songs about trains, cars, farms, and love… lost.

At a time particularly desperate, he was forced hide his truck and tractor in his neighbor's machine sheds in order to elude bill collectors. To his name, all he could claim was a small pile of rosewood scraps, two blank cassettes, and a friend named Willie P. Bennett.

Fred hit "record and play" on the old Panasonic. He and Willie played and sang to the built-in microphone. I'd give the tires off my truck for a copy of those tapes.

BILL STORK

Brothers Louvin and Everly sing in voices tighter than the DNA that binds them and richer than foam on a Guinness draught. Harmonious ain't the first word that comes to mind when Willy and Fred conspire. Willie's voice and mandolin stands behind and to the side of Fred, like the big brother who'll kick your ass. Willie's off-kilter echo of "There are some roads, I wish I'd traveled" underpins the angst of Fred's lament of a woman "he wished he'd never known" like the midnight dream when you catch your next breath. No less bloodcurdling than when Mary Clayton stepped up, clenched her fists and melted the microphone screaming "rape, murder are just a shout away" behind Mick Taylor's apocalyptic guitar line on "Give Me Shelter."

Fred and Willie recorded ninety minutes of original songs then drove to town to play on the street corner for tips in a tin can. When they'd sold the rosewood box and cassette tapes, they bought more cassettes and played until they had enough money to book a road gig.

Fred's monologues on everything from border crossings to Buddhism are Seinfeld funny. He is not, on the other hand, known for writing happy songs. "Well the phone broke the silence, like the screamin' of a siren" he laments a love looking to prove just how strong that she could be. "I just stare through the door screen, watch the cars come down the pike, their lights against the sky like a drive-in movie." The rest of the world gets on with their lives, oblivious.

"Son, would you help me on this platform, I'm not so good at climbing stairs," he paints an image of a decorated veteran from "what they called the Great War" who comes to watch trains "darn near every Sunday." "Number 47, she's a good one, Number 63 sings like a bird, Number 29, that's the one they call The Rocket..." I beg you to buy the *Balin'* CD. If you can get from cover to cover with two dry eyes, *I* will refund your $16.95.

"I saw Big Bear Henry and Two Turtle Jim, rolling into town, they was riding on the rims, sold their tires to buy themselves a couple cases of beer," sounds like just another Saturday night in Decatur, Illinois, for Doug Quintenz and Dave Randolph.

Fred is never more desperate than "Rough Edges":

"Cracks in your windshield, holes in your life,
and you're tryin' to get home, before it gets light,
*and your **old five-ton truck** don't run good no more,*
barely gets up those hills with your foot to the floor."

The "old five-ton truck" that made an indelible impression on me sat at the end of a quarter-mile farm lane, forty-three miles east of St. Louis, high atop a ridge overlooking Shoal Creek, in 1974. It is the 1950s International stock truck on my Aunt Mary and Uncle Kelsey's farm. A bent piece of fence wire through the dash worked the choke. Three hard pumps and a Hail Mary and she'd back-fart, blow smoke and rumble to life. If you pumped the clutch and worked the wire just right, you could keep her runnin' first try. Burlap feed sacks covered the crumbling foam and kept the springs out of your ass where the white vinyl used to be. Two lids off an old hog feeder and four rivets kept your boots dry when you couldn't dodge the puddles. The struts that held the big bubble fenders had long since rusted away so they waved at the neighbors as we passed.

The chickens would run short on feed coincident with the bottom of Uncle Kelsey's last Mail Pouch long-leaf chewing tobacco, and just before hay was dry enough to bale. He'd tell Aunt Mary he was gonna "show Little Bill the town." The hills that Old Five-Ton Truck could barely get up were on Pokey Road, which formed a triangle between Pocahontas, Greenville, and Old Ripley, population 108. The two corners of State 140 and County 22 were served by Garver's Feed Mill and Rip's Inn. (She usually was.) Once he had regaled the mill on Vietnam, Nixon, and grain markets, we'd throw our two bags of layer mash on the end gate. Kelsey Dillman would kick the International into neutral and we'd tha-thump on the flat spots on the dry-rotted Firestones from the loading docks into an open spot next to the front door of the tavern.

We'd belly up to the crown molding rubbed raw by forty years of farmers' "table muscles." Kelsey would throw down three eight-ounce Budweiser drafts from just across the Mississippi, and I'd go toe to toe with RC from the gun. We didn't want Aunt Mary to think we'd been sittin' at the bar.

As a cross-tribute to my Uncle Kelsey, Aunt Mary, and Fred J. Eagle-smith, my three-quarter-ton Ram diesel wears the license **5-TON**. (A calculated misrepresentation, as the vehicle weighs barely 7,400 pounds.)

I'm expecting an email from the folks at Dodge darn near any day now. En route to down cows, we have punched through snow drifts higher than the hood ornament. One memorable Fourth of July, the trailer hitch became the saddle horn for the dead end of a halter rope. The other was occupied by a Red Angus heifer in hot dystocia and less than impressed by our efforts to aid in the delivery of her firstborn. I was back on the hard road after tubing a steer who had bloated on fresh green pasture, when the Sirius went silent. I had dropped into four-wheel-drive to gun it through a drainage ditch. An airborne hunk of peat bog had skewered the antenna.

Three hundred fifty days a year, the eight-foot cargo bed is covered with my mobile veterinary hospital. Under the full-length door on the driver's side are antibiotics, anti-inflammatories, sedatives, and stimulants. There is a one-cubic foot AC/DC refrigerator for vaccinations, a ham and cheese on wheat, or an occasional six-pack. Under the passenger side coffin door is room for gallons of lubricants, laxatives, vaginal progesterone implants, and two lassos. ("Bill, two rules: 1. Never carry a lasso. 2. Never learn to use it." — Dr. Fred Kuffel. Well Doc, I'm one for two.) Behind the tailgate is a drop-down door that accesses two drawers that fit rope halters, rumen pump and nasogastric tubes, a surgery kit, hoof knives, and an emasculator (as in the veterinary tool, not to be mistaken for an infamous ex). Space on the sides is perfect for garbage, recycling and a Stone Ratch-a-pull calf extractor (a tool that is particularly unsettling when presented to a birthing class full of rather sensitive first-time mothers at Fort Atkinson Memorial).

As for the remaining fifteen days a year, a guy likes to use his "pee-cup-truck," as Dr. Randy Ott used to faux drawl, for R&R. Twice a year we like to explore the splendors of southwest Wisconsin by horseback. This year, at Christmas, Paige asked if I could come and pick her up from college at the end of the semester, a question to which there is only one answer, though it requires some decontamination of the driver's quarters and removal of the Port-a-Vet.

Historically, Jason and Junior at Steve's Car and Truck Service have obliged. After the requisite grumblin' from the boss man, they always had a forklift that could pick up the 2,200-pound piece of fiberglass like the head off a dandelion, a good option that always left me feeling indebted, dependent and minus an hour and a half of travel time.

Presented with such a structural dilemma, all the son of an Operating Engineer needs is a scratch pad and John at London Lumber. With pen wedged under my Packers hat and wielding a twenty-five-foot Stanley retractable tape, I leaned across the counter and showed John that I needed to span eighteen feet and an eye bolt to hook a cable come-a-long. He looked out the window.

"How much does that rig weigh?" he asked.

"'Bout a ton or so," answered the son of a construction worker famous for his over-engineering.

I explained that the tack room was eighteen inches taller than the horse stalls, so I had to build a scab on the low side. I hoped the use of a carefully chosen construction term would temporarily disguise my outright ineptitude with a hammer and nails.

"Ya know, Doc, I bet if you put together two LVLs, that'd be plenty strong enough to pick that up." He leaned on the counter and calculated. "I'd have to make sure, and we'd have to order it in for you. How soon ya need it?" he asked, fully expecting that my lack of planning was going to cause an emergency on his part.

"First week in May," I responded. I would Google "LVL" when I got back in the truck.

"Ah heck, that's no problem." He promised to get back to me.

I left my number. Before I made it to my next farm call, the phone lit up.

"Yeah, Doc, I got two eighteen-footers in the warehouse. You want

BILL STORK

us to drop 'em off, or pick them up?"

I may someday *need* a favor, and I like to haul stuff. "Ah, don't worry about that John. I'll be by with the trailer."

London Lumber is 2.8 miles north of Cambridge, one block west of Highway 134. Just slow down at Febock's fallen-down barn on the east, and turn left at the London Oasis. Half the letters have fallen off the corrugated steel façade of what *looks* to be better spot for a haunted house. London Lumber does not Facebook or do "11% off on everything in the store." There is no need for an obnoxious pitch man or a catch phrase. They've got good straight lumber and guys who know how to use it.

It is said that no one exists in a vacuum. I have been influenced by truly exemplary characters, both blood related and brothers by association. When I wear my construction cap it is with the old man over my shoulder. If you're lookin' at a two-hour job you want done by Sunday noon, order the materials on Monday, lay out your tools Friday night and get at it by six o'clock Saturday morning. If two 3/8 lag bolts will hold it good, you use four half-inch carriage bolts with stainless warshers. You could probably pick up an eight-foot Porta Vet with one, but you just never know when a stray two-ton circus elephant's gonna go down on that very spot. You might as well double up and bolt 'em down good.

Experts say we begin to form associations in the womb. I struggled in high school Spanish, but thanks to the machinists, millwrights, mechanics, and carpenters who put their feet under our dinner table, I could qualify for an honorary Ph.D. in the vernacular of the workin' man. Former Navy Chaplain Father Bob just gives a nod and sentences me to a couple of extra "Hail Marys" when it ain't quite level and a carefully chosen exclamation is required to move that bubble between the lines.

It's funny how much smarter my dad is, the older I get.

"Don't jump off the tailgate. That back's gotta last you a lifetime," he'd suggest in the name of self-preservation. "Just because you can get daylight under it, don't mean you can lift it. That's what ropes, pulleys, and bucket tractors are for."

The vet box was in the truck, and it had to come out. When it came time to mount the massive laminated beams originally intended for a church steeple, I had an afternoon and Calvin. There comes a day when Dad grabs his son around the waist to invert him and do a pile driver, just to maintain pecking order... and the son doesn't move. It had been a year since that day.

I was fumbling with some ropes and chains, figuring how to lift the lumber on top of the bucket tractor without dropping it on my head. I looked behind me. Calvin had military-pressed and slid the south end of the 6'x10' by eighteen foot laminate onto the top of Boomer's box stall. The north end was taller, so I threw down two guard rail timbers to get high enough to sit on top the tack room.

We'd come up with a way to tell grandpa we didn't use the tractor later.

No job is complete without a little diesel smoke. With a homemade choker, I could get close enough to the tow hook on the bucket of the John Deere and lift the back end out with the tractor.

Circumstances and my limited construction chops have made these moments painfully few. For a seventeen-year-old man with little time with a ratchet in his hand, Calvin has some keen construction instinct. He had cut, drilled and bolted his end without checking his phone. Save the expletives, shims, and the Hail Marys, the eighteen-foot span was top-dead-center level, first try.

I backed the truck through the barn and Calvin gave me the "whoa" when the front eye on the vet box was directly under the five-ton cable ratchet lift. I slow-curled my fingers until he inched the tractor forward and lowered the bucket over the lift hook on the back. As I cranked the come-a-long, Calvin matched my progress with a steady hand on the lift lever, and the one-ton piece of fiberglass rose smoothly above the wheel wells. I pulled forward. In less than an hour, the 2014 Dodge mobile veterinary hospital had become a moving truck for a college freshman.

BILL STORK

With accomplishment comes a swagger. I didn't expect him to post it on Instagram, but I did want Calvin to see the Porta Vet hanging in the barn, and the truck drive away before he left for work.

The college freshman in question was, of course, my daughter, Paige. If asked to describe her in one word, it would be: thoughtful, quietly-competitive, compassionate, over-achieving and tolerant. With a father's objectivity and no regard for the overuse of hyphenated adjectives, I add selfless and soft-spoken.

At some point, Paige must have realized that she'd soon find herself facing twenty hours on the road with dad.

Knowing that early May is the vortex of the tsunami which is "busy season" at Wisconsin Equine, Paige asked, "Is there any way Sheila might come along when you pick me up?"

I could have *not* taken it quite so personally, until she added, "If it's easier on her to come earlier or later, I could skip a few finals or hang out on the street for a few weeks."

Anyone who has come to know me since October 2009 has Sheila Barnes to thank. Alma Ann Beasley was genetically incapable of putting her concerns ahead of an amoeba. In the process of calculating what *everyone in her sphere* needed, mom was paralyzed at the notion of making a decision. Dad was a construction worker. Something would be torn down, built, or fixed by 8:00 a.m. Monday through Saturday. Completing a sentence just cut into the work day. In the fifty-one years I've known him...

This apple would have been still sitting directly under the tree, lonely and rotten, had I not learned to expedite my communications.

Sheila to Bill: "Where do I show up? When?"

It could be a manifestation of opposite attraction or aspiration. While brevity is as elusive as organization for me, Sheila's claim to fame is bullet-point communication and efficiency.

Any given day, you'll find her wearing khakis at a Wisconsin Equine management meeting by 7:00 a.m., and in scrubs assisting a colic surgery in the afternoon. Saturday and Sunday mornings have found her on the wooden end of a fork stripping, pitching and spreading thirty box stalls when barn staff no-shows.

It is humbling to imagine how man *could not* have progressed were it not for the horse. They are noble, elegant, and athletic. Whether under saddle working herds of cattle, fighting wars and transporting mail, or in harness breaking ground and pioneering the West, horses are creatures upon whom man has been wholly dependent for centuries.

Horses have been photographed, filmed, painted and featured in cowboy poetry. Some advertise their love with tattoos, belt buckles, and blankets. Sheila with a horse is simply *at one.* Whether riding, working, trimming, brushing, feeding, cleaning stalls, or baling hay, she is at peace in the midst of her herd.

If I were *required* to describe Sheila in one word, it would be: accountable, an all-encompassing trait of which I hope Paige and Calvin can glean some fraction.

If an iPhone 5 ever implodes or melts down, it will be hers.

According to Google Maps, it is seventeen hours and thirty-five minutes from Cambridge, Wisconsin, to a spot in Vermont within clear earshot of a boulder-strewn mountain stream. The goal was to arrive with time for twenty-four hours of hardcore R&R before departing for The Green House at the University of Vermont. There we'd join the sweating parade of parental Sherpas negotiating bookshelves and papasan chairs around stairwells, as our environmental scientists and engineers retreated to the four corners for summer break.

Women will conspire, Exhibit A: Paige asked Sheila to come along to spare her eighteen hours in the cab with Dad. Presented with an opportunity to properly absorb nearly forty hours of my wit, wisdom, and barnyard philosophy, Sheila brought *seven* books on tape.

My Amazon critic Sarah accused me of being "stuck in the good old days." Looking to grow from valid criticism, I reconned our 1,037-mile route on Google Maps and synced it to my phone. It would give me turn-by-turn directions from my driveway to our little New England Bohemia.

There *is* enough old-school in me that I would be more comfortable with a Rand McNally in the seat pocket; you just never know when the satellites are simultaneously going to fall from the sky, or your battery go dead. It was T minus 8 hours before departure and I had five minutes for a quarter-pound cheeseburger from Kwik Trip and a mad dash through Walgreens. I've made it a game to come up with some obscure item to seek when I walk into Walgreens. The helpful young man at the first checkout knew the precise coordinates of the Midnight Jasmine nail polish; alas, he could not find an atlas.

I programmed the route from the Lake Mills Veterinary Clinic to the MK Cellular store, to confirm that turn-by-turn directions were "all systems go." Though she never hesitates to yell at me when I go off the grid, the lady in the phone who announces "Turn left in a quarter mile" had suddenly fallen silent.

Panicked, I burst into MK Cellular where Mark, Luke, and Cory have gracefully resolved every tech issue with no more than six key strokes and respect. I cued up the navigation app to demonstrate my problem, at which time the robotic wench announced: "You have reached your destination." They can't fix what ain't broken.

Afternoon appointments went down smoothly. By the time chores were done at home, dogs were loaded and gear stowed, we were "southbound and down" with a Subway steak and cheese by eight p.m. Our first goal was to get through Chicago and around the bottom of Lake Michigan. We'd drive until we were delirious. The farther we made it Tuesday night, the easier Wednesday would be.

No good story is without a sub-plot (or several). Gray and his Airedale were my second client, twenty-three years ago. In the quarter decade since, we have water skied from ice-out to December. As I write this story on a chair in my garage, I can reach out and touch a 100-ft. sixteen-gauge extension cord, a power strip, four laser lights, and his right-angle drill. I use his boat as if it were my own, in exchange for a half an hour in June and again in September. I think I may have loaned him my chain saw once, and filled a hole with my tractor.

Gray's mother is the embodiment of grace, strength, and dignity. Mother's Day was but a few weeks away and Gray wanted to create a water feature from a millstone. In the month since he'd asked, I had failed to procure one though I had asked every old-time tractor collector, and scoured ten miles of fenceline. In New England, 1722 is considered modern era construction. I would scour the roadsides, ditches, and antique shops; Gray would scout the interweb. If there was a millstone in Massachusetts, New York, or Vermont, it was coming home.

The 2014 Ram 2500 Diesel is a high-tech workhorse. It can pull a three-slot horse trailer without breaking a sweat. The dashboard looks like the cockpit of a Boeing 747. It has an eight-inch data screen, Bluetooth, and Sirius Satellite Radio. At an additional cost that we may have considered, it can also have on-board navigation. The in-dash CD player has gone the way of the eight-track, cassette, and three-on-the-tree, an observation I did not make until hours before departure.

In an effort to protect any chance at our future, Sheila showed up with an old-fashioned handheld player, on sale at Walmart for $9.99.

Three and a half hours may be enough time to dissolve the stresses of work if she had been at a rodeo, on the back of a horse, or the bow of a pontoon boat with a fruity rum drink in hand. Passenger seats are famous for inducing Sheila into surgical anesthesia faster than 20cc of IV propofol. On this occasion, however, she had yet to achieve Zen. I assured her that I had a cable to plug the player into the data port, though I had not actually visualized it.

Note to self: when the salesman asks to show you all the high-tech features of your new Dodge Ram... take the time.

If there is a time when Chicago traffic is a minimum, I rightly fig-

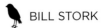

ured eleven on a Tuesday night would be it. We sailed through the north suburbs on the Eden and confidently onto the Dan Ryan. The Chicago Skyway/Route 90 was clearly marked and we hugged the shores of the lake and headed to Gary, Indiana. There would soon be three states of smooth sailing. Before Indiana mile marker 12, I-94 would wander off into Michigan and I-65 would go south to Indy. I was looking for I-80/I-90 to continue east.

All I had to do was follow the signs or the directions spouted by my phone.

At that exact moment, Sheila was far less concerned with our geographic coordinates. The carefully programmed phone was part of the debris flying about the cab as, in an extremely atypical moment of frustration, she continued to look for the elusive data port. Far less violent, but significant nonetheless, was the torrential rain that made a mockery of the wipers. Forty-five mph crosswinds were less of a concern as I found myself nestled among a convoy of fifty-three-foot tractor trailers. Secure as it were, the signs were but a blur as I struggled to find the fork in the roads.

There are times to speak; there are times for silence. In the name of self-preservation, and looking to maintain the sanctity of our little getaway, I chose "B."

Images of her laugh lines, dimples, pale blue eyes, and flaming locks of hair buoy my soul when times are low. She is defined by her common sense. The fiery temperament alleged to ride the same gene with red hair is largely lost on Sheila Barnes; frustration is usually detectable only by a Doppler blood pressure monitor or a skilled psychologist. On those occasions of more outward display, and if I'm in some part responsible, I have evolved the practice of SASG: I don't change the volume, the radio station, the speed of the truck, and I offer no apology. Extend the courtesy of non-reaction, and she'll do the same the next time you're throwing scrap lumber around the garage. Soon as it's safe, she'll silently hand you the carpenter's level you've been looking for the past hour.

The shortest distance between two points is famously *not* a triangle. My fears were confirmed when the wipers cleared the windshield and the green sign came into focus: Detroit 275. I had made the first significant navigational error of our brief excursion. The silver lining is that it was during our 100-mile excursion through southern Michigan that Sheila was able to locate the elusive data port.

Truck-stop coffee, chocolate-covered espresso beans, and 5-Hour Energy: nothing keeps an errant traveler wired like the angst of knowing it could have been avoided. Sleep was not a thought until twenty-two hours after I had woken and we were back on I-80 eastbound.

Defeat could only come if we lost a single second of our twenty-four hours of R&R.

That ain't happening.

By eight a.m., the flipped-down visor keeping the rising sun out of our eyes, we had thirty-five gallons of diesel on board, a quart of 100 percent Columbian truck-stop mud, and a Little Debbie Danish as we merged onto I-80 East. I'd be no less honored to sing back up with Bruce Springsteen than to be on one of the busiest interstate highways in the U.S. running with the big boys and girls. It exceeded Dr. Stork's rough math to calculate the volume of freight between any two mile markers. If it gets imported, exported, eaten or built in this country, 70 percent travels by truck. To be nestled among the OTR pros doing their jobs buoyed my brain.

As the fertile croplands of Ohio gave way to the rolling dairy paddocks of Pennsylvania and Massachusetts, the sun traveled its daily arc from just above the visor to our rearview mirror. We weren't going to make it to the Long Trail Brewing Company before they closed at seven, and the Backyard Barbecue didn't open until Memorial Day weekend. Token and Remmi were road-weary. Bill and Sheila were toxic on pretzels, peanuts, and snap-peas. Hell-bent as we were to reach our destination, the 1846 Tavern and Grill was well worth the U-turn. Token and Remmi made the acquaintance of Buford the Basset, and we reclined in anything that was not a bucket seat, basking in the glow of the stone fireplace and pan-seared salmon.

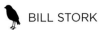

BILL STORK

Sheila and I would later reflect on Thursday May 7. We sipped coffee, speaking just over the din of the birds and gurgle of the stream that meandered beyond the mountain meadow. Token leaped through dead-fall as Remmi scrambled down the walk path. I set down my mug to carry her back up, only to find I had once again underestimated the old girl's heart. Breakfast would be leftovers from the 1846 over three eggs, and in no kinda hurry.

We hiked Deer Leap Lookout as Token scrambled up the rocks like she was born on the Appalachian Trail, hoping to go as high as the remnants of the record New England snowfall. Remmi guarded the truck. Just north of Woodstock and three miles down a postcard dirt road led us to Sugar Bush Farms.

Two steps into the kitchen, the lady wiped her hands on her apron and stepped away from waxing bricks of cheese. She shaved a microscopic sliver of smoked cheddar that was near nirvana (Grand Champion at 2013 World Championship Cheese Competition in Green Bay). We lounged and sipped Long Trail Ale as the sun set on what Sheila would later call "A Perfect Day."

Paige said she'd be ready to load out by late morning. It was a two-hour drive to Burlington and I expected traffic. A drive across Vermont is a feast of the senses; avoid the interstate except for emergencies. We arrived with enough time to walk the shores of Lake Champlain with Remmi and Token and listen to the howls of a homeless Rastafarian echo off the walls of a city administration building.

Loading Bill out of Lincoln Avenue Residence Hall at the University of Illinois, circa May 1984, required a three-quarter-ton Ford pickup truck and a twenty-three-foot stock trailer. Dad had built bunks that hoisted our beds to the ceiling, leaving floor space for a Davenport and a trundle bed. No dorm was complete without the requisite beanbag chair and bookshelves. Once my neighbor introduced me to Stevie Ray, and Kish indoctrinated me into the school of Van Morrison, the Panasonic with built-in cassette and receiver with turntable patched in would not do. A poor college student couldn't justify or afford a respectable stereo, unless it was a pair of Klipsch Horns with a 200-watt slave and a pre-amp to control it. Then he could book small DJ jobs. It became a source of income, and new CDs (released while I was an undergraduate) were tax deductible.

Loading Paige out of The Green House at the University of Vermont, circa May 2015, required three trips. Her gear would have fit in the glove box of a Smart car. Her goal is to be able to carry her belongings on her back.

I treasure every day I get to spend with Paige and Sheila. There are moments of frustration to be managed. You'll recall this entire journey is underpinned by a conspiracy that we'll refer to as "The Muting of Dad." They will smile softly and look dismissively just past me. They claim to know what I am *really* thinking.

The unspoken accusation is: "Dad is thinking, 'If we have a full tank of gas and lunch on board when we pick up Paige, then we can beat traffic over the bridge back to New York by 1:30. With a quick rest stop at the Welcome to the Empire State, we can go hard until a late supper in Ohio. If Remmi is doing okay, we can be back in Wisconsin in time to mow grass Saturday morning, go for a bike ride, catch the early band at Tyranena and then the Cash Box Kings in Madison at the Crystal. With a seven-minute nap, I should be up by five on Sunday to get three hours of writing done.'"

Those thoughts *never* crossed my mind.

So, when Paige asks apologetically, "There are a few things I'd like to check out before we get going," I soften all body language.

"Oh sure, Paige, this isn't a race. That would be fine."

Translated, "Dad's in town with the MasterCard."

It is a rare day the famous Farmhouse Restaurant in Burlington does not have a two-hour waiting list. In anticipation of 450 miles of Ohio-Indiana deep-fried tollway poison, we sat in the shade of the umbrellas on the sidewalk while the free-range, all-natural, organic calf that would eventually grow up to become the steer that is humanely laid to rest in order to become one of the most creative twenty dollar hamburgers I've ever eaten was *weaned*.

BILL STORK

We made it through the Patagonia store for a bit under a dollar a minute. Surrounded by two hundred dollar high-tech, performance rain coats, a twenty dollar ball cap is a bargain.

Paige disappeared into the Outdoor Gear Exchange. The uber-helpful young sales rep inexplicably asked if I needed to know where the bathroom was as I deftly rifled through the closeout rack looking in futility for an XLT, and rocking from left to right.

I thanked her and asked, "You wouldn't happen to have a road atlas, would you?"

"Dude, that is so totally old-school!" as she pointed to a rack next to the climbing ropes.

U.S. Interstate Highway 80 runs 4,000 miles from the Hudson River in New York City to the San Francisco Bay Bridge. It is always four, and at times up to eight lanes wide. I may someday be able to reconcile having lost track of it once. Twice in four days, and I'd demand my father write me out of his will, present myself for castration, or both.

Paige and Sheila sorted hammocks. I camped under a modern art sculpture on Church Street, oblivious to the patchouli and body odor, studying the atlas.

I'd take I-7 South out of Burlington to Route 22. I had seen the signs for New York on our way into town. Route 22 would turn into 17, and take us across the lake. I didn't need to know the highway that paralleled the lake to the south. I'd just follow the signs to Ticonderoga, where I'd take 74 West to Interstate 87. That would deflect us a bit south, but I calculated our speed of travel would compensate any extra distance. In no time there'd be a sign for Akron, I-80, and a straight shot back to Gary.

In time, the girls emerged from OGE. There was no way to be in the shadow of both Ben *and* Jerry without going for ice cream, unless the line ran out the door, around the corner, and disappeared into Montreal. We opted instead for an elixir called Kombucha. Kombucha is evidently made from holy water blessed in small batches by Pope Francis and aged in golden urns. It comes in a variety of flavors and is available at City Market, a popular UVM store that strictly prohibits BGh, antibiotics, and antiperspirant. They require armpit hair and pay their employees a stipend in proportion to the percentage of their body covered in tattoos.

In demonstrating to the girls just how relaxed I can be, I attempted to be unaware of the time. We made it back to the truck, exercised Remmi and Token, and I glanced at the digital clock on the dash. Half-past four, only thirty minutes later than my most generous estimation. With some efficient navigation and keeping rubber to the road, I could get both yards mowed Saturday afternoon.

I was basking in my brilliance as the Green Mountains gave way to a fertile plain populated by CSAs and dairy farms. We topped our tank at the Addison General Store, which had a pump with rolling numbers, seven dollar Vermont ball caps, and fifty pounds of ribs in a smoker out back. We were headed south toward the home of the lead pencil when Sheila asked, "Do you want me to cue up the navigation on my phone?"

At the risk of undermining my confidence, "Sure," I said. "I've got a pretty good bead on this situation, but it never hurts to have a backup."

I have perfect recall of the intersection of I-87 and NY 74: I had swung wide and depressed the signal lever that Sheila so boldly accuses me of neglecting, when her phone spoke, "Continue forward on Route 28."

I hesitated, but assumed that Google Maps was straightening out the southern reflection of 87. In doing so, we would take a two-lane trip through the wooded lakes of the Adirondack Mountains. Bonus.

We found a vacant ballpark next to Long Lake. Bladders were bursting, and Remmi and Token were ready for a romp. We lapped the outfield twice and had a team meeting. Given our time frame, there wasn't so much to see between Upstate New York and Cambridge, Wisconsin. The Rock and Roll Hall of Fame would surely be cool, but locked up tight at one a.m.

BILL STORK

Paige hadn't driven a car in six months, but she's a gamer. She volunteered to take a shift behind the wheel. Sheila, if you recall, is famous for vehicle-induced comas. I envisioned myself taking the two a.m. to home shift.

In the Dodge Ram commercials, the little girl is giggling from the backseat as she watches the foal race the Quad Cab down the gravel drive. As my underloaded, three-quarter-ton Ram chattered over road construction and lane changes, the fifty-year-old guy in the jump seat is less amused, my bald noggin bouncing off the windows like a bobblehead in a paint shaker.

I sat bolt upright as Sheila navigated, "Okay, Paige, take 190 North."

Leaping from broken sleep to tachycardia, in my mind I traced the route from Burlington to Cambridge; we should *never* be northbound. In less than a quarter of a mile we were on the brakes, having joined a one a.m. traffic jam that looked like Black Friday at Walmart.

Behind the glare of the green and red lights, I could make out "Bienvenue au Canada."

The iPhone asks nicely if you'd like to avoid toll roads. Clearly, foreign countries are no big deal. The shortest route between Burlington, Vermont, and Cambridge, Wisconsin, is straight through southern Ontario.

Paige spent three weeks in Peru at the foot of Machu Picchu when she was fourteen years old. She ventured to Finland for a month. I expected that errantly arriving at the border of our friendly neighbor to the north and being fluent in "hockey" would cause her less stress than "Where's the ladies room?" Feeling responsible, situationally castrated, and a bit surprised, I rolled down my window.

The only passport among us was buried in a garbage bag under the tarp in the back. We were the fourth load of under-documented travelers misguided by technology; but we were surely the first who displayed their loyalty to Fred J. Eaglesmith on the license plate. (Remember Fred?)

I was certain the border guard would notice the "5 TON" homage immediately. Recognizing our declared allegiance to their poet laureate, they would offer a free pass, if not an escort across the Province.

I waited for an opening.

The guard presented us with a 3x6 piece of scrap paper and pointed us to the glass building. Well-armed and hyper-friendly Canuck number 2 explained that while we were more than welcome to travel through Ontario, he could not assure our fate upon re-entry.

Feigning casual, I rocked back and laughed, pointing to my truck.

"What's so funny?"

"Ahh," I said, "how ironic that I find myself stranded at the border, only ninety kilometers (switching to metric should seal the deal) from the birthplace of Fred J. Eaglesmith."

I waited for the offer.

"Who?" he seemed puzzled.

"Fred Eaglesmith," I repeated. "White Rose, Indian Motorcycles, Cumberland County... you know, *that* Fred," assuming that repeated exposure to Jake brakes made it hard for him to hear deep voices.

Nothing.

I looked around to see if there was a supervisor available. Clearly, I was being vetted by the only Canadian who did not know the significance of Fred. If there was another official, he'd whisk us right across. The Buffalo, New York, border crossing is not exactly crawling with people in the wee hours. He pointed to the gate that would open as we approached it and explained the route back south.

Back home, I reflected. Had I taken two more steps and ten minutes at Kwik Trip in Lake Mills, an atlas would have fallen on my head. If I had pulled over to follow the one I bought in Burlington at the intersection New York 87, we wouldn't have been able to save all this time to swing through Michigan and bounce off Canada.

BILL STORK

Leave it to Sheila to pick up on one small detail. "If you had a license plate on the FRONT of your truck, maybe the first border guard would have been a Fredhead."

Maybe it was best I encountered the only two Canadians who didn't know Fred. Fred's border crossings are not uniformly flawless. If there is a vehicle that raises more suspicion than a three-quarter-ton truck, it would be a twenty-five-year-old bus smelling like french fries, driven by a gravel gut student of Buddha in a stove-pipe hat and a pinstriped tuxedo with tails. Mysteriously, Fred's Traveling Steam Show is prone to inspection. On at least one crossing, Fred's Bluebird had been detained. His guitar player, Matty Simpson, was found with a half-dozen expired roman candles.

Next time I align myself to a Canadian in expectation of amnesty, I'll try Ann-Margret, Sarah McLachlan... or maybe Pam Anderson.

Free Bird

If I live to be a hundred, or tomorrow never comes, I pray that my last memory will be sunken in an over-stuffed chair on a cold February morning, 1997.

Paige felt medium-rare, lying across my chest. Flaccid, except for the shiver at the end of each inhale, her head lay lifeless against my neck. In her heaviest fleece footie PJs, zipped to the top, she was swaddled in a quilt and draped with my twenty-year-old, red-checked Woolrich.

No radio, TV, or computer. I sat silent and aware of her every breath. Like Buddha meets Big Nutbrown Hare, exploring the length, breadth and depth of a father's love for his daughter. This moment delivered by a simple cold that in due time will pass, while internalizing the anguish of families for whom the entire world was reduced to the child on their shoulder, suffering from cancer or incurable disease. Dogs, cows, and accounts receivable would wait.

It could have been five minutes or four hours, but in time, the twenty-pound radiator on my chest cooled. She lifted her head, and whispered, "Bup."

In my thirty-two years, I had never known a greater emotional excursion from heartache to joy. I wrestled from the chair, letting blanket and flannel fall to the carpet. Cradling her with my right arm and pouring from gallon jug to sippy cup didn't leave a free hand, nor did I have inclination to wipe the tear as it fell to the linoleum. I pulled the tray and lowered her into the high chair.

For the rest of the day we watched videos and read stories: *The Giving Tree, James Herriot's Treasury for Children...* and *Thea.*

 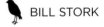 BILL STORK

The pages of the book about a little tomato who was not like the rest were dog-eared and tattered. Twelve years later for an English composition class in high school, she burned the message forward to the pubescent crowd, and a lawyer, electrical engineer, and an insurance salesman to whom I emailed it.

She wrote an unapologetic essay demanding our society own up and not sweep literature like Huckleberry Finn under the rug so that we can continue to move further away from where we have been. Her children and generations to follow should have the opportunity to read history in the language that it was written in.

With one ear trained on a circle of adults waxing on social issues, a sixth-grade Paige pulled on a tube of strawberry Gogurt.

"I think we'll see the day when it makes no difference when a black person applies for a job," I said. Pleased with their sensitivity, the adults paused.

"I look forward to the day when we describe people by the color of their shirt," Paige quietly applied the exclamation point... with a velvet sledgehammer.

Paige knew the story of *The Giving Tree* by heart and by blood. We had read it a hundred times or more; it could have been written about her grandma. Dementia would siphon her soul years before fever took her life.

In order to know her namesake grandmother better and in hopes of sparing another family the devastation of dementia, she knocked her dad from the perpetual cycle of "I oughta" and "I wish I had." Paige rallied the family. On a cold, gray September Sunday morning, we marched across the John Nolen bridge over Lake Monona, shoulder to shoulder and eye to eye with caretakers, victims and families in the Walk to End Alzheimer's.

Her thoughts are exponentially fewer than her words. What once appeared to be lack of motivation to an oblivious dad, we would learn years later was an excess of pride. Defined by the notion that "not all who wander are lost" and driven to see the sun rise over Machu Pichu, Paige found her own employment en route to an underserved school in Peru. In doing so, she taught her dad that faith is a powerful tool, and God isn't the only one who deserves it.

She is strong enough to play hockey with boys more concerned with hitting one another than passing the puck.

She is the picture of contentment, reading a book at sunset over Taylor Lake, Wisconsin. Her wanderlust carried her to the fjords of Finland, shrinking the globe to her family at home, and providing experiences minimum wage could never buy. Spending summer in a country that speaks little English, has never heard of barbecue sauce, and is an easy bike ride from Mother Russia.

With two cans of Yuban on sale and a box of corn flakes, I waited my turn at the Cambridge Piggly Wiggly. Contemplating the tabloids: Jen's latest break-up and J-Lo's surgery. A hearty handshake brought back reality. Two proud dads on a Sunday morning relived a play-by-play from the "2009 Pumpkin Classic" – a cross-field pass that would have been a team gold were it not for a driving rain and vicious cross wind that was equal to our girls' valiant effort.

In five years that feels like two ticks of the clock, our daughters are about to graduate high school.

"What's Paige up to?" Curt asked.

My spine jolted to army erect and pulse accelerated to 100-meter sprint. A sensation of inflation erupted in the chest – every last alveoli stretched with 100 percent oxygen, like two cool hands laid gently on my face, pulling my eyelids until they gape. I gathered myself quickly and shrugged, lifted my chin and turned my head. It was a thinly veiled attempt to hide the heart I wore on my sleeve.

"She's graduating near the top of her class and going to the University of Vermont…" emerges from my lips, while I think of the seven-year-old girl who scored three goals in one hockey game. She could not get past the gauntlet of parents and out of the boutique rink at Madison Ice Arena fast enough.

I think, "Over-accomplished and insanely concerned about the feelings of others," but "She is doing really well, going to school in Vermont next year," I respond.

BILL STORK

From their cradle to our grave, we agonize over every action, reaction, and decision, hoping that our kids only have to look across the dinner table for a role model, so that when they cross that stage and turn their tassel, they are stepping from bedrock into the unknown.

Standing in the introspective crosshairs, in one moment thinking the paradigm has shifted hard, then realizing it is truly a symbiosis. The daughter for whom we walk the line is the force that reminds us who we are.

With subtleties of family and friends, her core is uniquely and beautifully Paige. She did not invent independence, accountability, compassion, or strength, but has made them her own.

Thanks to the little girl on my shoulder, I'm more aware of my carbon footprint, considerate of the person behind me, and slow to critique what I don't know. We can bold it in all caps and write in red ink on five-dollar Hallmark cards. We hug them and step away, emphasizing every superlative with clenched fist, and crescendo to a pregnant pause: we are so unbelievably, phenomenally, enormously... P-R-O-U-D.

Admiring who she is, I pray to live long enough to see who she becomes.

I Ain't Never Had Too Much Fun

It was nine o'clock on a sweet spring evening as we sat around the firepit. My son Calvin asked for ten dollars so he could bowl a couple of games.

I enthusiastically responded, "Sure!"

He dropped his head, and then his shoulders. I pointed to the concrete pad, minus the one-car garage that once stood over it, covered with three-quarters of a load of split oak. His ski buddy, Tim, was with him.

"With two of you and the tractor, it should take about a half an hour," I continued. "Paid in cash, free from deductions, you'd be doublin' your money from the DQ."

"You just don't care about having fun, and besides, you could make that money in ten minutes," was the less-than-calculated response from the otherwise intelligent young man.

"You just don't care about having fun." Those words would set into motion a hundred miles of "phone-on-the-dash, radio off" kinda thinking. With my fiftieth birthday within shootin' distance, this was not my first negative performance review.

I have evolved the notion that when presented with a criticism, embrace it. React for as long as you must, ignore the context, dispense with the excuses and internalize the validity within their words.

If you should find yourself sharing tea and Triscuits with Attila the Hun who points to his mouth, then don't talk with food in your mouth. If your boy says you work too much, you ought to pull up a stump and put your chin in your hand.

BILL STORK

A fine piece of barnyard pop-psychology, if I've ever written one.

Like a Bo Ryan point guard who just committed a turnover, the boy was about to get ten minutes on the bench and a talkin' to. I have worked really hard to never start a sentence, "When I was your age," mostly so my kids could never accuse me of saying, "When I was your age." I'm pretty sure I've adhered to the rule; they might roll their eyes. The choice to verbalize his frustrations bought Calvin an impromptu lesson in economics 101; macro, micro, and veterinary.

My barely controlled diatribe was void of profanity, save a few "softies" for emphasis. I began by describing driving west on Highway 16 in September 2007; he was eleven. I listened in horror as the newscaster broke into U-2's "Pride in the Name of Love" to chronicle the near crash of the stock market. My odometer read 200k, fuel gauge below a quarter tank, and his sister Paige was seven years from starting college. It was all I could do not to pull over and deposit my breakfast in the ditch.

Calvin's biggest concerns at the time were showing his work on his multiplication by the partial sums method, and playing hockey from St. Louis to Minneapolis. Meanwhile, the adult-type folks were scrappin' hard just to keep our nostrils above water.

"You can make that money in ten minutes," said Calvin.

We went on a field trip from the firepit to the driveway. I dropped the end gate on my old Dodge and pulled out a pile of clothes. Tide may get out the dirt KIDS get into, but an hour face down in a calving pen will leave a guy explaining to Dodge County's finest as to why you're driving home at one a.m. in your boxer briefs. My Pella green coveralls were supersaturated with placenta, blood, and enough manure to make the Maytag man turn tail.

I dropped the wad on the blacktop with a splat. "I made ten dollars in ten minutes, at midnight, last night lying face down and armpit deep, pulling a deformed calf from a cow. How was your night's sleep?"

"Not to mention, I spent the better part of ten years cleaning dog poop out of stainless steel cages and pig piss out of Smiley hog feeders at a rate of ten dollars *per half-a-day* in order to earn the right to do so." (Notice the artful omission, yet obviously implied, non-use of "when I was your age.")

At the time of this little father and son chat, he was still sporting the "goggle tan" from a week of spring skiing in Breckenridge. I did some "dad math." If he had to try and cash flow his skiing career working eight hours a week making Blizzards, he'd be afoot, just short of Omaha.

I could not help but invoke the all-encompassing wisdom of the Web Wilder Credo: Work hard, rock hard, eat hard, sleep hard, grow big... and wear glasses if you need 'em. I'm no dairy farmer, but I am not prone to sitting around or backing down from a double cheeseburger. I couldn't find my backside without my bifocals and 36x34 britches strike me about mid-ankle.

I reminded the boy that on the days designated for fun, I played second fiddle to none.

For the past twenty-five years on a given September Saturday evening, the population of otherwise peaceful "Stork Valley" swells a hundredfold. Barbecue, pork, and brisket waft amongst the laughter of kids on the Joust House and zip line (largely thanks to Calvin, who chaperoned for two hours last year). Big city attorneys have their manicured hands engulfed by farmers known as much for their friendly demeanor as their third generation dairies.

As the sun sets on the whole scene, the barn radio stuck for a year on "Outlaw Country" gets drowned out by a W.C. Handy award-winning Old-School Chicago Blues Band. Dad's sore knee saunter turns to west coast swing, and the Red Wings work boots are dancin' shoes.

As I watch the budding oak leaves split the morning rays, there comes a revelation. There are three generations of Storks I can personally account for, and we have a requirement. Whether you are hunting, fishing, cutting firewood, or putting a roof on the neighbor's garage, you're at it by sunrise. I don't mean thinking about putting the coffee on, fryin' eggs, or on the throne with last Sunday's comics.

BILL STORK

I grew up with, and adhere to the notion you can never catch a fish lest you have a line in the water when the sun cracks the horizon. It also does not matter if the fence line you're clearing for firewood or hunting rabbits out of is in Brazil. You leave early enough to get there, get your guns out or sharpen your saws by sunrise.

What Calvin and I didn't know is that things come around like clockwork, once a generation. Sitting at the dinner table under the genuine oil reproduction of The Last Supper with my parents, I had asked, "Can I use the truck tomorrow night?"

Not for lack of trying, I had no girlfriend. At 6 foot 3 and 165 lbs., with hair Ronald McDonald red, my chances were dramatically improved in The Brown Bomber. The Bomber was a 1976 three-quarter ton Ford. She was spotless with metallic brown paint polished four times a year, an orange accent stripe, and aluminum mag wheels.

"Sure," Dad responded, between bites of meatloaf and gravy, "soon as it's empty."

It was sitting just outside the dining room window with nothing more than a tool box, a log chain, and a come-a-long, but that's not what he was talking about. Sixty miles south, our 5'2" carpet-layer friend Jim Adkins, who farmed for relaxation, had a fence-line that was overgrowing a bean field. As soon as those volunteer elms and box elders were cut, split and stacked under the pine trees in the back yard, I was free to address the date deficiency dilemma.

I'm pretty sure I was no more excited about spending a day cuttin' and stackin' wood than Calvin was spending half an hour. The thought of complaining never really crossed my mind. Some days Dad said we're cutting wood; some days we fished.

A decade later, clearing trees on the lot where we would start a family of our own, I paused to fuel and oil the Stihl Super 028. Dad had bought the saw after I barked my shin with our old McCulloch. I had violated the first rule of felling a tree, but it didn't have a back stop. He wasn't keen on spending eighty dollars for the nice Korean doctor at the country hospital in Shelbyville to put sixty-eight simple interrupted sutures in my knee. In addition, he needed an explanation for Mom as to why it would never happen again.

I looked west over Korth Park and thought of a dead apple tree in a friend's back yard in Decatur. I had a hatchet you could shave with and a homemade guard of cardboard and duct tape. The handle was red from the head to the grip. A generation or two before had worn the handle to bare ash. Dad ran the chainsaw. He put the tree on the ground, right between the chainlink fence and the telephone line. I stayed ahead of him with the hatchet, taking out the small branches and keeping his feet clear.

Somewhere past my twelfth birthday, I still had "ten and ten" and had swung the hatchet long enough to clean the branches tight to the trunk and chunk the brush up small. The firewood stacked straight as a game of Jenga, and the brush pile lit with one match and a Sunday paper.

As Dad was halfway up the trunk of the gnarly old apple tree, the saw went wuhumph… like it had been thrown in the lake. Out of fuel. Class was in session. Chainsaw 101: always start it with your foot through the handle, never cut toward yourself, make sure your feet are clear and always fill the bar oil when you fuel. Dad put the old yellow war horse in my hand, and pointed.

He picked up the hatchet and went to work. A tap on the shoulder reminded me to keep the butt of the saw low, and cut away from myself. With a creased brow and a wave he reminded me not to pinch. My feet disappeared under the shavings, and Dad was dragging brush and loading logs.

As I shook my head clear of the memories, finished my Dr. Pepper and started back to work, I sighted down the naked trunk of the white pine. Twenty years on from the apple tree, I realized Dad could have cleaned those little branches that I had hatcheted in a breath with the chainsaw.

Even in my warmest memories I would not use the word "fun," but those were the days when you didn't question. Parents will get mad at their kids. We are well served to filter our fury through the realization that in so many cases, it is knowing that we have let them down.

BILL STORK

What my dad did for me is to draw a clear line between "Dad said so" and a day on the lake. Decades later, in trickles and waves, the lessons learned in the woods are still washing ashore. Feeling a chainsaw chew through an old dead apple tree would have been only half as sweet, had it not been for a couple years on the hatchet.

Calvin is a free-style park skier. A Misty 540 or a K-fed filmed on a buddy's Go-Pro and posted on "you gram" will get him 200 hits.

Throwing the saw and bar oil between the stacks in the bed of a three-quarter ton Ford squattin' on the overloads will give you a perspective for life.

Dad climbing into the passenger seat, and the sound of a 460 four-barrel growling through the hollows of Southern Illinois, tugging six cords of winter warmth, will square up your thirteen-year-old shoulders.

Twenty years on, you realize it's kid earning and dad bestowing... trust.

Wrapping the truck and trailer in the corner of the gravel lot and slapping the sawdust from our jeans and boots is not exactly frat boy fun. Yet to this day, I recall the double cheeseburger and Coke "from the gun" at Mugshot's Bar and Grill on County Highway 11, between Cowden and the Kaskaskia River.

An accomplished artist and potter named Rick LaMore once said, "Following your dreams is a noble notion, but it makes damn thin soup."

We all have to spend a lot of time doing what we have to en route to the things we want. If we learn the reward of a lawn mown clean and trimmed tight, or a cow fence straight as a sunbeam and solid on the corners, the white lines between fun and work will forever merge.

Calvin, as for the accusation that I work too much: guilty as charged. Being known as a hard worker is admirable. Being defined as such is dangerous. Only being comfortable when you're productive is pathologic. Let's go golfing.

Every Dog Has His Day

There once was a day when I nearly thought I was cool. It would fly in the face of my very nature to make such a blanket statement. More accurately, cool by association, and for brief and fleeting moments in time.

Then I had teenagers.

By virtue of genetics and vocation, I talk a lot. Had she lived until the cell phone, my mother would have stricken fear into the heart of Mark Erdmann at US Cellular and his unlimited minutes and data plan, like the Green Bay Packers showing up for All U Can Eat For $6.99 Buffet at Denny's.

As veterinarians, we practice medicine and surgery, but one of our most valuable products is information. Not to mention, I am a big fan of language spoken well in any form. I live to hear Wayne Larrivee broadcast the Packers on Sunday afternoons, but I'd tune in if he were doing play-by-play of a house being painted. My Chicago friends would laugh 'til they cried at the notion, but I used to listen to the traffic report from Madison. Sure, it was roughly the equivalent of a backup at the one stop sign in Mayberry, but I emulated the cadence and diction of the gentleman who reported. I try hard to speak accurately, if not succinctly. (Thank you, Sheila.) It's a work in progress.

I've even been corrected by my daughter.

I had just seen a high school friend. "Hey Paige, I ran into CT Taylor at the Kwik Trip in Lake Mills, he's a professional long-drive golfer." She rolled her eyes and curled her lip like I had farted on

BILL STORK

the Maitre d' at L'etoile. "Dad, you know you just doubly identified the topic of that sentence." Guilty as charged.

It may have leaked out that I like music. It is a significant point of pride that I have hosted Joel Paterson, Oscar Wilson, and Joe Nosek in our barn. Collectively they are the *Cash Box Kings*. These young men are not simply the keepers of the blues, they insure the art form and culture will continue to grow for at least another generation. Joel has been called a freak, a genius, a magician and the "best guitarist in the city" by the *Chicago Tribune*. He has quietly commanded the attention of purists all over the planet with his multi-track, one-man homage to Les Paul, Chet Atkins, and Merle Travis, called *Handful of Strings* (available at Amazon and CD Baby).

One of the most memorable nights in Madison music history came on a frigid January night at the Crystal Corner Bar. The legendary Wayne "the Train" Hancock had found himself without a band. His guitarist and steel guitarist had rendered themselves unable to perform in an epic artistic dispute that became physical. JP shook hands, plugged a pawn-shop hollow-body Gibson into a seventy-year-old tube amp the size of a carry-on, and proceeded to level the joint. Playing songs he had never heard with a man he'd never met.

Oscar Wilson has fathered a dozen children, survived cancer – twice – and is a museum piece. He grew up on the south side of Chicago; his father died of cancer when he was nine years old. In his place were Muddy Waters, Buddy Guy, and Junior Wells, who would sip iced tea, eat his mom's fried chicken and play the blues on his back porch to pass the sweltering Sunday afternoons.

In 1980, John Belushi bravely predicted that by the year 2006, "The music known as the blues would exist only in the classical records department of your local public library." "Joliet Jake" did not know about The Big O. When Oscar sways to the microphone, you don't know what he's about to do; the band has not a clue. The only thing for certain: it will be Old School and it will be blues.

As things started to come together for this year's version of our little gathering of friends and musicians, my son Calvin interrupted without looking up and asked, "You're not having that old-time hillbilly crap again this year are you?"

For a father who has shared fewer suppers and sunrises with his kids than he had hoped, I find myself counting. My daughter Paige is starting to pack her bags for college in Vermont; her return to Wisconsin is no more certain than Peace Corps in Peru. Calvin is fewer than 700 days away from graduation. The only thing I would bet on in his future is mountains and snow. Wisconsin has only one of those.

September through May, we find ourselves the voice of reason…

"Calvin, I can't help but notice a zero in pre-calculus on January 24," I pointed out. After a bit of thought he responded, "That's the day I took my driver's test," as if that were all the answer I should ever need.

"Calvin," I asked, "did you expect Mr. Uhen to take the day off and watch movies in honor of your passing behind the wheel?" No response.

In my experience so far, thirteen-year-old girls and sixteen-year-old boys respond in one of two ways: deadpan or not at all. "Calvin, what did you do all day Sunday?" I asked reasonably.

"There was a rail-jam at Alpine and there were two Olympians there," he responded with a month's worth of energy.

When I asked about the looming AP European history exam on Monday, he responded as obvious as a Clydesdale on your toe, "The lifts close at seven."

June, July, and August we pack it up and put it away…

In the eyes of a teenager, adults are categorically uncool, "You're not wearing that in public are you?" With eyes that have aged since my last prescription sunglasses, I turned my hat backwards to get close enough to the dashboard to read the gauges: "Dad, if you're gonna wear it backwards…"

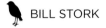 BILL STORK

We look for hooks. Until this year, I thought I had it made.

June 18, 1992, was a Thursday. I know that because it was my fourth day at the Lake Mills Veterinary Clinic, and I confirmed it on Google. The eight a.m. appointment was an Airedale terrier who thought he was a Corriedale sheep. Having grazed his meticulously fertilized back yard, he found himself what you might call "bound up." I was new to town and looking to make friends and connections. The owner, Gray, was as tan as the dog's curly brown coat. Once Moose was pooping like the geese that denude his lawn, I asked about the trailer hitch behind his Chevy Blazer.

"What do you pull behind that truck?" I asked hopefully.

"Barefoot Warrior Supreme with a 250hp Yamaha," was the equally enthusiastic response.

With regard to ski boats and friends, there tends to be a dynamic. I like to think of it as symbiotic. Those who have boats need help putting in piers and lifts. Unless you're Bugs Bunny playing baseball, you cannot by definition drive and ski at the same time. Those who make the payments may call the same relationship parasitic. Ahh, semantics.

I stuck out my hand and responded, "I have three five-gallon gas cans and can drive in a straight line." We exchanged numbers, and twenty-two years, three kids and two boats later, we are still friends.

In the early '90's, we once pried the proprietor of boat storage from a stool at Moe's. The ice had come out early on a leap year and we were bent on being able to stake claim to having skied Rock Lake in February. There are pictures on the wall of Laker's Athletic Club to show that we also braved six inches of snow and driving winds to claim the month of December, and prove definitively we had not a lick of sense.

Then, in February 1996, my daughter Paige was born.

In the past eighteen years, we have spent far more time behind the wheel than in the water – teaching our kids and their friends to get up on a pair of skis. The thrill of watching your daughter rise effortlessly out of the lake on one ski is exponentially greater than a barefoot beach start or a slalom course run at '38 off.

If there is a sensation greater than sharing a passion with your children, I can't conceive it.

There are faux-antique signs for $19.99 at every marina and gift shop within skippin' distance of any body of water: *"A boat is a hole in the water into which you throw large sums of money."*

The Stork Corollary would follow: *"A boat is a hole in the water from which you extract memories."*

Having been on the receiving end of a fortunate father for my first twenty-eight years and a generous friend for the last twenty-two, I have never made a boat payment.

I learned to ski behind a sixteen-foot aluminum Starcraft with an 85-horse Johnson outboard, under the instruction of what had to be the most patient man ever born. I carry a thread of guilt that teaching me to slalom ski cost Wayne some measure of his seemingly endless sanity. By eighth grade, I was big enough to pull the boat around the lake and aim it where I wanted to go, so we up-sized. The "Cat Dancer" was a twenty-one-foot inboard-outboard, just smaller than a Mississippi River tugboat, but not quite as agile.

Recall the nature of my dad and the ease with which a construction worker is dislodged from a blue collar dollar. She had a motor that was darn near silent, except for the ticking of the lifter in the third cylinder. Repurposed from a Singer sewing machine, you were not going to pull a ten-person pyramid in the Tommy Bartlett thrill show.

While some boys ogled girly magazines, I pored over advertisements for Ski Nautique, Mastercraft, and Malibu in *Water Ski Monthly*. Occasionally we would get a glimpse of one across Lake Shelbyville. The notion of ever driving, or God forbid, skiing behind such a craft... unthinkable.

The boat that my kids would learn to ski behind had no such limitations. The 1994 Malibu Echelon looks like a fighter jet without the wings. Powered by a fuel-injected 350 borrowed from a Corvette, she could pull the Tommy Bartlett pyramid on their bare feet. At slalom speed, she throws a wake so polite it never breaks the sizzle as you carve an edge from one imaginary buoy to the next.

BILL STORK

Technology before its time. Pick a speed, program the Perfect Pass cruise control, and the speedo needle would never move. Twenty years of meticulous maintenance later, she looks like the day Gray pulled the plastic off the seats.

From Paige giggling uncontrollably, riding an inner tube in her swim diapers at idle around the lake, to Calvin's aerial 180 on the wake board last year, the Malibu did it all. For a half-dozen Tuesday afternoons in the summer time, I had 'em... or so I thought.

I have known some amazing intellects: Kishan Khemani, Dick Bass, and Arlin Rodgers, to name a few. All have become productive and respected in their fields. My son Calvin, adjusted for age, is as smart and intuitive as any. Let me go on record as saying that if his ambition and entrepreneurship ever synch with his taste in life, there are no limits. If you ever find yourself wondering the MSRP and standard features of a Lamborghini Aventador LP 700-4 Roadster, Calvin is your go-to.

Recently, we took Paige to a restaurant in Williams Bay called Pier 290. Looking for a spot on the lake to celebrate her amazing effort through high school, I was unaware the restaurant was also a boat dealership. On sight, Calvin began to rattle off the stats of each of the boats. I was blind.

He pointed to the Mastercraft X-Star. Each boat is designed online to your specifications. Capable of hosting a Catholic family reunion, standard features include a sound system out of Alpine Valley Music Theater and underwater lighting effects synched to the stereo. In ninety seconds it can pump up to 6000 pounds of extra water in order to throw wakes custom designed for shape and size by the onboard computer system big enough to host long-board surf competitions. Options include on-call professional instructors, massage therapists, and nutritionists. Models available only in California come with drones and a video production crew. Twenty-six feet long from bow to stern, it requires a Peterbilt semi to haul it to the lake, and costs more than my home and clinic.

Calvin knows these things not by memorizing the website; his friend Thomas has one.

One of the finest boats in its day and an old school slalom skier, I feared the Malibu and I may have gone the way of the Radio Shack TRS-80.

The text came Monday at midnight: "Can I bring a couple of friends?" Tim, Thomas, and Calvin are known to travel as a trio; Stooges they are not.

Along with his sister, it would make a boatload... of fun. Tim is oversized, overaccomplished and understated. He is the least experienced in tow-behind water sports, but a gamer. Calvin and Thomas will issue detailed instructions from the boat, and I quote: "Huck it 'til you feel your feet," or "Just weeble it." On no more than three tries, Tim was hucking and weebling.

The cheerleader of the bunch, Thomas could sell a Brett Favre jersey to a Bears fan. At home, Thomas' family's MasterCraft X-Star features a king-sized memory foam mattress and a bidet, so you never have to go ashore. At last count, he had wakeboarded twenty-one consecutive days behind the most advanced boat made on water. Yet I could have pulled out a piece of barn siding with ski boots, and he'd let out a war whoop, pump his fists and ride it.

Clear a piece of schedule, and commit to an afternoon on the lake and you are guaranteed that something is going to break down, it's going to rain, or the wind's gonna blow. Tuesday, July 8, we were fortunate: the boat ran great, there was not a drop of rain and no one got hurt, but the wind did blow. She blew all day with half the ferocity of a derecho, but ten times as persistent.

Dad fought to find the calmest water on the lake. That turned out to be about 150 yards along Shorewood Hills Road, where we dodged two sets of grandparents doing figure eights in their runabouts, with two or three grandkids in inner tubes giggling behind.

The boys were oblivious. They rode every piece of equipment in the boat 'til Thomas could stand it no more. Polite by nature, but deciding that even without the ballasts, computers, and professional groomers of his Mastercraft, the Malibu wake would do just fine, he asked, "Do you know anyone who has a board I could borrow?" A couple of text messages and a trip across the surf to a friend's personal pro shop, and the boys were in business.

George Berkeley famously asked, "If a tree falls in the forest..." you know the rest.

Bill Stork asks, "If a boy jumps two wakes or does a 180-degree wrap and no one is there to film it on a GoPro, SnapChat, Screenshot and post it on Facegram, did it really happen?"

Two "Ts" and "C" may never know.

For hours, Paige quietly watched and I drove, minus a couple of breaks to "check the temperature of the water."

With half an hour of daylight left and their stomachs starting to growl, the boys could huck and weeble no more. Yet, leaning quietly next to the motor cover was one piece of equipment that had not been in the lake today. Since the '40s, lake rats have experimented with countless versions of the personal hydrofoil: a way to glide silently above the choppy water below, and break your tympanic membrane or turn your eyelids inside-out while reacquainting with the water. The Sky Ski was the product of eighty years of engineering and the brainchild of an amiable old California surf-bum hippie named Mike Murphy, with financing courtesy of King Hussein of Jordan. (Yes, really.)

The Sky Ski is all over YouTube, but in the interest of time, imagine a short fat waterski with a milking stool on one end and a pair of sandals attached to the other. Extending thirty-six inches below the milking stool is a thin aircraft aluminum strut. To the bottom of the strut is attached a hydrofoil... like an airplane wing.

The pilot slides his feet into the sandals, straps the milking stool firmly to his backside and takes the rope in an overhand grip. On signal, the boat driver gently pulls. Once out of the water, the rider instinctively pulls the rope to his waist and leans back. Like a dolphin in the surf, the foil comes out of the water, carves a perfect semi-circle above the rider's head, and he or she crashes.

Finding their third or fourth wind, the boys were intrigued. Tim had never seen one, Thomas had a half-dozen but had yet to ride them, and Calvin had ridden once. Being the most experienced, he volunteered to demo. Suddenly thoughtful, having nothing to do with his crop of goose-bumps, the setting sun and the freezing cold lifejacket, Calvin suddenly perked.

"Hey, Dad, you've been driving all day, do you want to show these guys?" he bargained.

When your son asks to play catch, the answer is yes. Though it felt a little like the first dance to the last song of the night, I climbed out from behind the wheel.

It took no time for me to be in the lake. I strapped in and signaled Calvin to go. It had been a few years, but it took minutes to get the feel and speed dialed in. In the boat, Paige and the boys huddled under blankets and towels and struggled to stay awake.

The key to the Sky Ski is to keep it on the water at first and don't forget there is an airplane wing attached to, and three feet beneath, your butt. Keep your weight forward and your hands high. Gradually lean and lower. You will rise gracefully above the water, which brought the mummies in the boat to sitting upright.

I gathered a measure of confidence from this, and sliced from one side of the boat to the other, porpoising in a controlled fashion from the surface of the lake to the top of the three-foot strut.

Calvin circled his head with his index finger to indicate a turn and I followed the boat. By the time he found the next straightaway, I had the setting sun over my left shoulder and some mojo. I pulled hard to the port side and let the Ski slow to a stop. In a momentary lapse of reason, I cut hard to the wake. As it approached, I dipped the tip, dropped my hands, and heaved like pulling a hip-locked bull calf from a Jersey heifer.

Fully at the mercy of Bernoulli's equation of fluid dynamics, I heard a *Whaawoof!* on the percussion of water rushing to fill the space I had just vacated.

With the grace of a pterodactyl, the fifty-year-old bald veterinarian was airborne.

Twelve feet above the lake, I sighted down the rope. The boys looked like the front row on the Screamin' Eagle, with their mouths in big ovals as they threw off their wraps and scrambled for iPhones and the GoPro.

If I hadn't fully thought through the launch, I had contemplated the landing even less. As the apex approached, the time was nigh. The pucker factor was off the scale, precluding any chance of involuntary enema. For the cameras, I would maintain a poker face, like it was all part of the plan. As for the landing itself: weight back and a Hail Mary.

As the splash settled, Thomas jumped out of his seat and karate-chopped like I had just done a 360-degree tomahawk jam to win the state championship. It is a rare day indeed when a dad can be cool enough to be featured on his kid's GoPro.

Pleased and hungry, I cut and jumped for a couple more passes.

There is a reason Chuck Berry never wrote a song longer than 2:30. I tapped my head to signal I was done and sank into the water. As Calvin circled, I half expected to return to fist bumps and high fives.

Owing either to the famously brief attention span of youth, or because under NO circumstances is a dad allowed to be cool, I pulled myself onto the teakwood deck to the fanfare of a piece of driftwood.

Doc, Come Quick!

On any given day, "Doc, come quick as you can!" are not the first words you hope to hear. Especially shouted into an answering machine by a frantic farmer at two a.m.

Laurie Wright continued, "don't even bother bringing your calf puller, this one's gonna be a C-section!"

I have acquired from my brothers Scott Clewis and Kishan Khemani an appreciation for the romance of baseball and a taste for curry and wine with names I can't pronounce. But in my adult life there has never been a question of paternity: legs that would embarrass a spent laying hen and the ability to sleep under any conditions are genes that could only come from my father.

There are pictures of Dad, his Manitowoc Crane hat pulled over his eyes, dreaming of eighteen-inch crappie while leaning on a post at San Francisco International Airport. While anything but silent, we Storks are versatile, skilled and efficient in slumber; capable of achieving Rapid Eye Movement sleep medically indistinguishable from surgical anesthesia in a fraction of the time it takes a Starbucks barista to craft a triple venti half-sweet non-fat caramel macchiato at 120 degrees F.

Wake us from that sleep, and you are on your own.

Just ask Naishad Shah.

Naish is an electrical engineer. Currently he is in charge of synching distribution for McDonald's. Order a Quarter Pounder with cheese Extra Value Meal from the drive-through in Lake Mills, and there is a cow from Australia and a bag of potatoes from

Idaho headed for Wisconsin.

Naish is slightly built, brown-skinned, wears his polyester pants just under his armpits and dances like Pee Wee Herman. He could design a fully functional space station from your scrap iron pile and an old trolling motor. Notice I said design – you're going to build it.

I've known Naish since my freshman year of college. He graduated with honors from the University of Illinois in about thirty-six hours and took a job with IBM.

Needless to say, it was fully out of character to get a call from him on my dorm phone at three a.m.

"Bill, this is Naish." He seemed a bit anxious.

Oblivious, I answered as if I had been up for hours, "Oh, hey Naish. How you doing?"

He did not return my pleasantries. "Bill, I'm in jail and I need some help."

As if he were asking to borrow a cup of milk for his cornflakes, "Sure, Naish. Whatcha need?"

Naish had come back for a reunion and to visit his brother. In no time the reunion became a group of ten of us, excited to reconnect with our friend and do some networking. It was an excellent opportunity for us to learn about life on the outside. There was also an unwritten rule: take a job and come back to visit = buy your poor college friends food and beverage.

George Chin's Chinese restaurant violated every single one of "Bill Bryson's principles of road dining." It had the yellowed plastic back-lit menu with indistinguishable items 1-86. Located on three levels in the middle of a college town, it was famous for a drink called the Volcano. Known by different names at differently themed bars – fish bowls, pond water, paint thinner, dirty bath water – drinks in that genre feature somewhere around twelve shots of various rotgut two-dollar liquor and food coloring. The Volcano was served in a pawn-shop ceramic bowl with faux pineapple trees and hula girls painted sloppily on the side in garish glossy paint.

From the middle of the bar protruded a basin the bartender filled with moonshine or turpentine and lit on fire. Consumed out of the basin through foot-long straws, around high-top tables, one sip of the swill is enough to raise your ALT 150 points and induce hepatic insufficiency. By the second, you will flatly fail a field sobriety test.

So the happy band of reunited Indian engineers cleverly had ten bowls. The "Hick" had a donut date with the Amazing Dick Bass at six a.m., with horse stall duty to follow, so I had a Budweiser, enjoyed the company and called it a night.

Driving was out of the question, even if they could have found their car. Instead, Naish made his way back to Florida Avenue Residence Hall to sleep it off in his brother's room. Under the circumstances, the numbers and doors all looked the same, and no one answered a polite knock on his first guess. Having exhausted his options and with an impaired ability to navigate, he chose to harmlessly curl up on the couch in the student lounge. Or so he thought.

When the residence advisor on night patrol discovered the unidentified Indian, he asked for an explanation. Incapable, or consciously choosing to take the fifth rather than implicate his brother, protocol required campus police be called.

Betty White would have been a greater physical threat, so they opted not to summon the SWAT team. Still, the campus boys lacked detention facilities and called in the city police. Experienced and trained in the ways of random vagrants and leaving nothing to chance, they took him and they booked him and gave him a quarter to use the telephone. (Name that song quote and win a prize. Arlin Rodgers is not eligible.)

Once he had been processed, printed, and stripped of his belongings, he found himself standing next to a payphone holding a quarter. Use it wisely, else a first time offending engineer risk the fate of Rubin Hurricane Carter.

Which brings us back to the phone call, twenty-five years ago.

"What do you need, Naish?" I asked, ready to leap into action.

 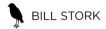 BILL STORK

"Eighty dollars!" he begged.

I remember the conversation as if it were yesterday. "No problem. I'll be right there."

As if I had so much as the proverbial pot, and knew where "there" was. I was a junior in college who bought his clothes from a store a store called Huey's that looked like Farm and Fleet meets Goodwill, and drove a 1974 Plymouth Valiant with plastic seats and an AM Radio.

Recall the thing about Storks and their sleep. Just as I promised my friend I would be right there, the telephone receiver hit the cradle, and my head hit the pillow.

It could have been hours or seconds later, but the very next thing I heard was the door slam. Kish burst in like a linebacker hitting a blocking sled, "Hick, wake up. Naish is in jail!"

I sat bolt upright in bed, clueless and shocked at the very notion. "Naish is in jail? What are we gonna do?"

"We need eighty dollars for bail money," he said as he went to douse his head in cold water so as not to end up cellmates. He had been at the same dinner party.

"No problem, Kish," I said. A big Indian at the foot of my bed and a small one using his one call from jail is not the norm for early Sunday morn. Yet, it was not the alarm to which I pledge allegiance.

Kish pulled the door shut, and I hit the pillow with a thud.

In retrospect, the whole scene had to look a bit like my favorite episode of the Dick Van Dyke show. Dick had been hypnotized to fall asleep and wake again on the ringing of a bell. Woken from a dead sleep by neighbor in need, frantically pushing his doorbell, as he made his way from the bedroom to the front door, the phone began to ring as well.

By the time Kish had toweled from the cold shower, changed clothes and drank a gallon of water, my alarm sounded. I rubbed my eyes and stumbled from my room to the scene of a half dozen

Indians draped over the living room furniture.

"Hick, where's the money?"

"Sure Kish, I've got six bucks. What's up?" I said.

"What the hell do you mean, what's up? Naish is in jail!"

So, we have a legendary ability to fall asleep, and an established history when that sleep is broken. Let us travel 250 miles north and fast forward six years, to get back to Chuck and Laurie Wright's poor cow.

I didn't own a heart rate monitor in 1994. If I had, I'm sure the thing would have exploded as I went from dorsal recumbency, R.E.M., and snoring like Paul Bunyan to "Come quick, it's gonna be a C-section!"

At the time I lived in one of those old farmhouses that had settled a bit. From the foot of my bed to the stairs, she sloped nearly imperceptibly. Drop an orange from the fridge, and it'll roll out the back door. The porch was the perfect place to watch the sun rise with a cup of coffee, but the rusty metal lawn chairs were all shimmed to keep your head rocked back while reading the Sunday paper. The garage was at the bottom of the hill from the house. All of this to say that once you woke up and found the floor, all you had to do was pull on some britches and keep one foot in front of the other. You didn't have to be awake until you got behind the wheel.

As the sandhill cranes fly, the Wright farm was less than a quarter of a mile straight west over two drumlins and 120 acres. Rather than drive cross-grain over plowed fields and line fences, I'd take the northern route. After 350,000 miles on one clutch (yup, braggin' just a bit), the Vortec V-6 in the '91 Chevy heavy-half pretty much shifted herself. Switzke Road was darn near straight and in the two miles north to Highway B, I had just enough time to gather my senses. In a half mile west on County B and the same two miles back south on Wright Road, I had mentally sequenced surgery kit, clippers, chains, bucket, and iodine disinfectant in the

BILL STORK

order they'd come off the truck.

Driving onto the Wright farm was a bit of an art form unto itself, requiring no fewer skills than the impending surgery. Pulling straight in was a city-boy rookie move that would leave your hood lower than the tailgate, and all the drawers in your vet box would fall shut before you could get your tools out.

A good cradle-Catholic veterinarian would find himself reciting a few extra Our Fathers and Hail Marys come Sunday morning, as you were obligated to back down, pulling past the farm by two lengths. As the front wheels broke the crown of the road, you had to spot the cinder-block corner of the milk house on your driver's side mirror and the concrete retainers on the other side. In gear and off the clutch and throttle, so as not to break into a free-fall on the loose gravel, you cranked your wheels hard just past the milk pump exhaust pipe, thus completing a reverse pee-whistle and landing on the flat spot, leaving enough room to walk around the whole rig.

With mind still reeling and heart still racing from the urgent phone call, I found my marks and idled down. As the passenger-side mirror scanned the retaining wall in the darkness, I saw the red-tip glow of my surgical assistant pulling on a Marlboro.

Chuck Wright sat with one leg on the wall and one on the gravel, in Johnson Creek track sweatpants and old leather high-top basketball shoes, no laces and the backs broken down into slip-ons. The white cotton dress shirt, long since relegated to barn duty, flapped in the light breeze.

As I rolled down the window, he turned his head politely to exhale. He rubbed his belly. "Yep, Doc, she went ahead and had it on her own."

Without a hint of acknowledgement, he continued, "While you're here, I've got one with a sore foot and a pregnancy check."

It has been said that actions speak louder than words. Evidently lack of words are deafening. I was only able to manage a grunt in response to Chuck's attempts at talk about the weather and crops. By the time I finished carving the abscess from the Holstein's right rear hoof and pronouncing the heifer bred, he had stopped trying.

I scrubbed my boots and stowed my gear. Standing in the open door with one foot on the running boards and one in the gravel I asked, "Chuck, what did you feel when you reached in that cow that made you think we were gonna have to do a C-section, for her to then calve on her own twelve minutes later?"

"Aw, Doc, we didn't see her," he explained.

"We were sleeping with the window open, and she let out a beller like I ain't *never* heard before."

Private Gillespie

Living among future engineers and doctors for eight years of college, the son of a construction worker and a stay-at-home mom can only absorb so much book learnin'. For the middle years at the U of I, Saturday mornings I merged with the Amazing Dick Bass at Ye Olde Donut Shoppe to graze on run-of-the-mill pastries and drink pond water in a porcelain diner mug.

While nutrition may not have served the four food groups, the wisdom of the "regulars" was well worth $3.50 plus tip. A fifteen-minute diatribe on politics, gas prices, or the erosion of family values from a retired blacktop foreman and a pipe fitter perched on red plastic stool at a dingy white counter felt like gospel. It would put a guy right back home at Mom's dinner table with Dad and neighbor Bob.

Our Saturday morning summits concluded by 7:30 sharp. Dick was months away from defending his Ph.D. in electrical engineering, which is enough to put most folks six feet under. Yet in keeping with his moniker, Dick Bass would ride his beach-cruiser Schwinn to a job site where he spent the weekend wiring and hanging light fixtures in Habitat for Humanity homes. He said it made his head hurt to squint over Zener diodes all week in the lab; made him feel useful working with some big "wors" and helping folks out – a tradition he had started back home in Georgia when Jimmy Carter started the program.

I would hoof it eight blocks south to the large animal ward at the University of Illinois College of Veterinary Medicine. There I cleaned box stalls for wild-eyed Arabian horses. Referred by their regular DVMs rather than treating them in the field, they were more inclined to kick your head from your shoulders than be grateful for dry bedding. There was a six-month-old Hereford steer who would pin me to the concrete wall given a chance. As bottle calves, it's cute to wrestle. The game changes dramatically when they outweigh half the U of I offensive line.

Every six weeks or so, I'd ask my boss if I could be a half hour late the following Saturday. Surprised that student help *ever* showed up on time, let alone ask permission to take a spa day, he would grin and grunt.

The hours for King's Barber Shop were etched, clear and permanent, in the glass at the bottom of the door:

8:00 to 5:00 Monday-Thursday
Open 'til 6:00 on Fridays, noon on Saturdays
Closed on Tuesday

It was less than five minutes from the donut shop to the barber. On nice days I'd sit on the bench and read the Daily Illini under the two-foot barber pole. Feeling the neighborhood come to life, occasionally I'd drop the paper and ask permission to pet the dog walking his owner past.

I'd keep the paper in front of my head as the screen door fell shut on the little clapboard home next to the shop. You'd first hear the porch steps creak, then the wooden heels of Wes' wingtips grow louder as he quick-stepped down the sidewalk. I sensed the squint behind the temple piece of his wire rims.

"Morning, Duroc," he'd greet me.

"Morning, Mr. Gillespie." I'd shake the paper.

In the time it took me to read the scouting report for the Illini vs Northwestern road game, he stowed the sandwich he carried in a brown paper sack and hung the jacket that had been draped over his forearm, trading it for a freshly dry-cleaned light blue smock. He would pull the zipper to his chin, flatten the collar and face the mirror to ensure his tie was straight. He would select just the right comb and scissors from a jar of disinfectant, dry them on a fresh white towel and tuck them in his left breast pocket.

BILL STORK

Brushing his hands as he strolled to the window, he turned the sign to "Open." Looking to ensure I was first in his chair and not exhaust the good graces of my boss, at the sound of the wood bumping the picture window, I'd rock forward off the bench.

Paper stowed in my armpit, I turned the knob and pushed the oak door past the spot where it scuffed the hardwood floor in a six-inch arc. The tinkling brass bell announced the first customer of the day and the cast-iron closer pulled the door back to the sticky spot. I waited and hunched it the rest of the way.

Just past the door stood a hat rack polished by generations who had come before. Arranged neatly on a glass end table were wrinkled copies of *In Fisherman*, *Outdoor Life*, *The National Geographic*, *Time* and *Hoard's Dairyman*. The reading material nicely bracketed the shop's demographic, but served as little more than props for the patrons who were there as much for the enlightenment as to get their ears lowered.

His pants creased crisp like Frank Sinatra, with surgical precision he deftly clipped, shaved and pontificated. When Wes Gillespie and his customer faced the full-length mirror, they would talk in hushed tones about wives, girlfriends, and kids. When he turned his chair and cleared his voice, the periodicals would drop. The topic of the day could be farming, foreign policy, or fishing. Wes knew of what he spoke, either gleaned from one of the magazines on a slow morning, or one of the many professors he coiffed.

Wes was the kind of guy you were proud to know, and even prouder if you could impart some wisdom to. Just above the doorway to the restroom hung a five-pound largemouth bass. A handmade barnwood Gone Fishin' sign on the far wall left no reason to ask about closed on Tuesdays. I would always try and talk to my dad the Friday night before a haircut.

"You know Wes, Dad caught a nice mess-a-crappie just off the point in Sand Creek last Saturday," I'd relay.

Short of my mother's arms, I can recall no place more comfortable than Wes Gillespie's red leather barber chair. As I approached, he'd turn it towards me. I'd settle in, planting my boots on the shiny, angled foot rest, tempted to hunker low so the little man didn't have to reach. He'd pull a wooden stool over and wave the barber's cape like a matador, settling it over my shoulders as he snapped it gently around my neck, placing a finger to ensure proper fit.

"Tight on the sides, flat on top," he'd say.

"Yes sir," I would respond, as if he had to ask.

If he didn't sense a big morning rush, he'd find the middle of my temples. With his thumbs he would press firmly, giving way to radiating circles. Eventually he'd stroke my scalp with all ten fingers from my brow to the base of my skull. For ninety seconds, midterms and lab reports were of no concern.

I'd snap back to conscious at the sound of the cool lube spray and the clippers snapping to life.

There were no guards or guides. The Andis pro-model clippers growled through my sideburns like a Sears & Roebuck riding mower. Hard as it may be to believe now, I once had a head of hair that Rosina Butler referred to as "chef salad." It may have been her awkward eighth grade attempt at flirting, but I was not amused. I heaved my sack lunch at her, promptly landing me in the hallway explaining myself to the assistant principal who had been standing right behind me.

The mop was not dissimilar in color and texture to the ill-mannered porcine I tended at the Swine Research Center. A fact Wes had deduced either by keen sense of smell or grooming one of the graduate students I worked for, and how he came to call me Duroc. (For those who have never worked at the Swine Research Center, a Duroc is a breed of pig that is red.)

Wes' clientele trended toward, but was in no way limited to, the utilitarian sector of a progressive university town. He tamed the manes of ag students and faculty, ROTC members, and Asian graduate students. As skilled as Wes was as a barber, his true talent was his ability to weave his clientele together as one. In the space of three questions, he could find someone you both knew. You only sat next to a stranger once, and usually only for a moment.

A function of artistic license (and an extension of human nature) is to take an event observed once and assign it as a character trait. Wes was repeatable to the point that King's Barber Shop was a regular stop when friends came to town for football games and campus tours.

A card carrying member of The Greatest Generation, Wes had only one story when asked about the flag on his lapel, and it was not of his own bravery or service. Having landed in southern France, he crawled between the tracks of a tank as Allied Forces advanced on Yellow Beach. Dodging German fire, a young soldier dove under the tank with Private Gillespie. As the tank paused between explosions, Wes strained to see the name badge and introduced himself to Audie L. Murphy.

If you stayed on the same page of *Hoard's* long enough, he cued up the story of his first job after WWII. Having grown up on a dairy farm, Wes was one of the first generation artificial insemination technicians. Long before technology allowed us to extend and store semen in liquid nitrogen, bulls would be collected in the morning and their semen chilled and filled in penny balloons.

With an extremely limited shelf life, distribution was by way of open cockpit airplanes. A dozen units of Brutus' Best would be dropped by parachute attached to a Thermos jug to inseminators waiting on the ground. To this day, I feel marketing gurus missed a prime opportunity.

With their viability waning by the minute, Wes was charged with the responsibility of getting the sperm to a recently ovulated cow. In the late '40s and '50s, facilities were not what they are today. There were days when dodging Nazi fire seemed a decent option when a herd bull was not keen on having his virility undermined and his girls violated by a perfect stranger.

Finally, Wes would roll the cape off my lap and deposit the clippings on the floor. I'd drop my chin as he folded my shirt under and applied hot Barbasol to the back of my neck. He'd pull the straight razor from the towel and across the leather strop that hung from the left side of his chair, and then place his thumb as a guide under one ear and shave the stubble baby butt-smooth under my collar.

With head as still as a mannequin, I'd scan for anyone who might benefit from the answer to the question he had answered a hundred times.

"So Wes, when you gonna hang it up and fish full time?"

"Ah, I don't reckon anytime soon. Who remembers an old, retired barber?"

BILL STORK

Prius Pete

Three generations of flat-land farmers at the stump of my family tree and twenty-two years in service of Wisconsin dairy farmers have often rendered me enraptured with ordinary country experiences. A rural route the length of the Land of Lincoln straight as a chalk line, or Farmington Road riding high on a Jefferson County drumlin can be a six-sense overload.

A has-been, half-rate bike racer and the son of a long boom crane operator and fisherman is required by blood to live in constant awareness of the wind's direction, velocity... and character. Three weeks past the expiration of daylight savings time I found myself heading west on Dane County BB in hot pursuit of a down cow, waltzing in my mind as Jason Isbell mourned a high school classmate, "you never planned for the bombs in the sand, or sleeping in your dress blues."

Suddenly, my entire olfactory apparatus was saturated, from nostril hairs to frontal lobe. Incapable of calculating the loss of a loved one in another man's war simultaneously with the victory of a six-month battle against flood, drought, leaf hoppers, and root worms, I turned Jason to a whisper. Like pulling my palm across a snifter of fine single malt scotch, the aroma of earthen loam and peat flooded into the cab through the cracked window, along with an airy-cool hint of sand.

My eyes followed the prevailing northwest wind upstream until I saw what looked like stadium lights crawling across the field. A 200-horse John Deere powered a forty-eight-foot chisel plow, burying the stubble and chaff to decompose.

I clenched my fist and smiled, uttering a silent yes.

The first six inches of snow would fall by midnight. With 180 bushels to the acre safely in storage, he could be at Crawfish Junction treating his haggard harvest crew to burgers and beers. But next May, the rains may only give him a two-day window; another quart of coffee and fifty gallons of diesel fuel in November could be the difference between getting a crop in the ground or staring at a pallet of $500 per bag seed corn shrink-wrapped in the shop.

The NFC Championship game is decided in three hours. The winner goes to the Super Bowl, the loser goes golfing.

Raising a crop of corn takes all year. The winner borrows a hundred grand to buy seed and fertilizer, books his fuel for the next year and prays the Asian markets hold strong.

The cycle begins anew each spring. On Easter Sunday, we pour out of church, peel our jackets and feel fifty-seven degrees on our bare arms for the first time since September. Anxiously waiting for the snow to melt so we can golf and rake last fall's leaves, we all make bets with Kenny Setz as to whether this will be an all-time record for ice out on Rock Lake.

Meanwhile, Dave Schroeder is measuring soil temperatures and fretting.

The tractors are fueled, oiled, and greased. The planter is calibrated and ready. Put corn in the ground too early and it germinates poorly, rots and fails to emerge. Pass on an opportunity between May rains and risk not making 112-degree days to mature a crop.

And so went the spring of 2014. As a result of a painfully late spring, harvest time came and corn has been slow to dry down in the field. Mother Nature will dry corn down to 15 percent moisture for free. Wait too long and she will also dump six inches of wet snow on a crop before Deer Season (yes, capitalized as a proper noun; this is Wisconsin, damn it). Gavilon Grain will dry your corn from 20 percent down to 15 percent moisture for a dime for each percentage point. With markets at $3.33 a bushel at best, those fifty cents are the difference between a paltry profit, and loss.

BILL STORK

En route to the Haack farm, I met Dave Strasburg pulling two gravity boxes around the big curve by Topel's Trailer Park and Driving Range, bound for Vita-Plus. I took my right hand off the wheel, raised my thumb and waved a silent "git-er-done." Once he'd passed and out of sight, I gave a full-fledged, clenched-fist upper cut right into the dead space over the center console of my Dodge Ram. Last Sunday when Aaron Rodgers found Randall Cobb for a decisive third down conversion, Packers play-by-play announcer Wayne Larrivee maniacally threw his trademark, "And There Is Your DAGGER!" assuring a Packers win. After six months of ulcers, 700 bushels of corn safely in storage feels like no less a home team victory to me.

I asked Ryan Haack what he felt around harvest time. After an obligatory period of contemplation, he stared into a field of bean stubble south of their calf barn.

"I love the cyclicity," he said. "You start with a bare naked field in the spring, you plow, disk, and plant the field. You hold your breath for the first green to pierce the surface, then you spend the summer praying for rain to come and the fall praying for it to stop," he waxed.

"You can hear the crack of the cornstalks, even before you can see the combine gobbling them up. One day, ten-foot stalks stand like beacons in the harvest moon, rustling like the waves of Lake Superior against Bayfield beach. The next, there's nothing but a few dry leaves blowing across an empty field."

Ryan Haack, philanthropist, philosopher, farmer, and poet.

As it turns out, not everyone is charmed by the fall harvest.

Running just on time for afternoon appointments, I stopped short of the clinic's front porch to fish my ringing phone from my breast pocket, three layers deep. "What's happening, Uncle Ned?"

I answered in what I expected his standard over-jovial tone to be, though with a hint of reservation. Ned and I don't Facebook or text, and he seldom calls midday. When he does, you don't let it go to voicemail. Ned wakes every morning to three great boys and a beautiful wife, and is famously happy-go-lucky. He started the conversation off mad enough to spit a ten-penny nail through a two-by-four and finished just a little bit hurt, like somebody had stepped on a puppy.

Ned had delivered two gravity boxes full of corn to Gavilon Grain. Back at the farm, Herbie Altenburg napped in the cab of his combine, burning daylight, diesel fuel, and time as he waited to unload his hopper before the snow flew. In road gear and at 2200 rpms, a John Deere 4250 will go 19.5 miles per hour. Pulling two empty gravity boxes, one wiggle and you end up with a really expensive "yard sale" all over State Highway 12.

Much to the chagrin of one particular motorist, constructors in 1927 decided it would be more efficient, environmentally sensitive, and cost effective to route Highway 12 *around* Red Cedar Lake, rather than *through* it. As a result, there is a two-mile stretch just south of Cambridge that is not safe for a Porsche to pass an old lady headed for the beauty shop in a Buick, let alone a farmer on a mission.

Rearview mirrors don't last long in a cornfield, and backup cameras aren't yet offered on most gravity boxes. Hedging the shoulder is to risk rolling the rig into the ditch, punching a hole in a $5,000 tire or crushing a Corolla like an empty can of RC Cola when you blindly pull back on. Fully aware but with no other option, Ned and his John Deere in road-gear accumulated an eight-car entourage.

As the solid yellow line broke just past County A, cars peeked around to ensure no oncoming, and began to pass. They politely pulled well past the bow of the John Deere before drifting back into the southbound lane. Cousin Karen frantically waved and swerved like a middle school cheerleader on Red Bull.

Last in line was a smartly dressed, dignified-*looking* gentleman in a Toyota who we'll refer to as Prius Pete.

We'll assume Pete was waylaid for the entire two-mile stretch. Knowing he would never think to exceed the speed limit, even if the Prius could, his desired speed will be assumed at 55mph. Behind Ned he could only go 35.5 percent of his desired rate of travel. As a result Pete had 4.2 minutes unceremoniously amputated from his day.

BILL STORK

(Stork's rules of rough math are fully in effect; the numbers are rounded in such a fashion that he can do the math in his head and if questioned they will hold up to cross-examination. To this point, they have never been exaggerated to make a point.)

We can all agree that when a man has a plan, seconds seem like hours. Let he among us who has never pounded the dash and uttered a few of George Carlin's seven words cast the first stone.

However, at high noon, one week before Turkey Day 2014, Prius Pete was not yet in the spirit of giving thanks.

When Pete's turn came, he pulled into the space between whining lugs of the John Deere. He rolled down his window so as he looked up from his 2500-pound, four-cylinder hybrid into the cab of the twenty-ton diesel, Ned would know just how mad he was. Ensuring he had Ned's attention, Pete leaned into the passenger space, scowled, and thrust his middle finger violently at Ned.

Pleased that he had communicated the gravity of the injustice leveled upon him by the man who milks eighty-five cows, farms 150 acres of crops and feeds 150 people a day, he floored it, all 1.8 liters and both batteries whirring towards Fort Atkinson.

Pop country hunks in cowboy hats, cutoff T-shirts, and ripped Levis like to sing about pickup trucks, tractors, and dirt roads. Farm and Fleet sells a million John Deere hats to folks who wouldn't know a PTO from a GTO, and every beauty shop and bakery has a year's back-issues of *Country Living* magazine dog-eared and wrinkled on the counter.

But when it comes to frozen fuel lines, backwards calves, bloody knuckles, and sore backs – all before sunrise on Sunday – the farmer stands alone.

So Pete (as Merle Haggard almost said), when you're flippin' off a farmer man, you're walkin' on the writin' side of me.

Milk doesn't come from Pick 'n Save and bread from Panera. In order to get from their farms to our tables, somebody has to get a little shit on their shoes. Now and again, there will be a thimble of inconvenience, even for those who don't have to step off the pavement. The Prius may have the acceleration of a jackrabbit, but 50,000 pounds of corn does not start, stop or turn in the space of a Kwik Trip bathroom. He can't go any faster.

The mission of this piece is an explanation on behalf of farmers in general. As it turns out, Pete, the man you chose to disrespect a few weeks ago happens to be my first friend in the state of Wisconsin. He is a father, husband, brother, and an uncle. I love him as if we were born of the same mother, and I respect him. A saint Ned is not, though he does sing in the church choir.

He was up at 4:15 this morning. When I was twelve, I moaned when Mom made me pick up my dog's poop and take out the garbage. Ned milked fifty cows every morning. In the forty-two years since, Uncle Ned has been the father figure and drill sergeant for his niece and nephews, a United States Air Force Blackhawk helicopter pilot, a beautician, a union electrician, and a steamfitter. His sister worked two jobs to support them.

As an assistant coach, he has mentored all three of his boys and their teammates in tenacity, respect, and wrestling. As is the case on most farms, theirs is a model of family and interdependence. It is made possible by his wife Sarah, the herd veterinary technician, relief milker, calf-feeder, mother, and housekeeper. She is a college instructor, Sunday school teacher, and private pilot. She is also my daughter's godmother.

With their skillset and work ethic, any farmer in America could take a job in town, work five eights with health insurance and retire with a pension. Ask them. Some will tell you they love the independence or the pride of production. Others will say that's just what they have to do. But all will say that farming keeps them closer to their family.

To be frustrated to the point of action that you later regret is human: Ned's knee-jerk response would have been to dodge the mailbox on the right and crush the little hybrid like a raccoon having a bad day.

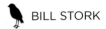 BILL STORK

Pete, please know that our purpose is not to delay your day.

If Pete is a lifelong cheese head, this surely was not the first time he shared the road with a SMV. If he grew up on the south side of Chicago, it can't be his first or worst traffic jam. It must require an astronomical accumulation of anger for a man to flirt with oncoming traffic side-by-side with a twenty-ton four-wheel-drive tractor just in order to extend his most demonstrative digit toward a damn good man.

So Pete, we sincerely hope that one day you can find resolution to the injustices that fried your backside, and for the well-being of those who love you.

Family Tradition

Traditions are like fingerprints: every family has their own. They are the twine that binds future generations to the elders. More traditions are focused on Christmas than any other time of the year. The infamous fruit cake with a half-life that would make a Twinkie seem like day-old bread. The two pairs of Levis my grandma bought my dad every year (the receipt would be taped to the box; they were always two inches too short).

There is an eighty-acre farm in northern Minnesota, seven clicks on Google Maps from the nearest four-lane, and eighty minutes from Fargo. It is defined by the ethic of the man who founded it and steeped in traditions that will ensure the family unit will forever endure, in daily ways that are tangible and timely. A cup of tea and cookie at ten and three pay homage to the physical toll and caloric demand of a farm that saw its first furnace not powered by chainsaw and splittin' maul in 2009.

Ways that are by definition never spoken and always demonstrated, in dire times can be the difference between celebrating a fiftieth birthday and a memorial service. Duane Schwandt's callused hands fit a hammer handle, saw, and tractor wheel for the hours each week it took to provide for his wife and four daughters. They were also there for holdin' and huggin' when one of his daughters or his wife needed it most.

Three hundred and sixty-four days a year, Duane saved and sorted scraps of kindlin' wood from job sites. Trees that overgrew fence lines and fields were cut and split to fuel the three fires that heated the well pump, water heater, and farmhouse. The brush was fash-

BILL STORK

ioned into a flammable tee-pee next to the pond out back where he'd use the 1948 John Deere B with a trip bucket on a pull-rope to clear a rink in the middle.

Christmas commenced midday with aunts, uncles, cousins, and kin playing broom ball, sledding, and warming at the bonfire. By the time the solstice sun would sink over North Dakota, the winter chill would wick the sweat from their waffle weave cotton thermals. En masse they would sojourn 100 yards up the field road. A foot of ice on a farm pond is anything but forgiving. Some were bruised; none were broken. The elders, anesthetized by brandy, limped and laughed, frozen to the bone. They would pile into the little farmhouse for a family Christmas feast and celebration of what they had: primarily one another and a pair of socks or gloves. If grain and milk prices were good and construction work aplenty, each of the four Schwandt girls would have a small toy.

On the days of the year that were not Christmas, life was not boot camp for Navy Seals. The girls were not allowed in the barn before school. To know the tenacity and interdependence of being raised a farm girl would eventually serve them well; the youngest would become head librarian at Jefferson Public Library. To go to school not smelling like a dairy barn was a significant point of pride.

It was also not catnaps and cartoons after school. The Schwandts milked twenty-six cows in wooden stanchions until a drought nearly wiped out the farm in 1976 and drove Duane to town to find construction work. As carpenters go, an artist he was not. Duane was the black coffee from a Stanley thermos jug craftsman who cut every corner square, planed every mantle level as an alpine lake at sunrise, and every door drifted slowly shut and latched.

On a farm ruled by example and expectations rather than doctrine, the Schwandt girls were allowed the freedom of band, choir, and sports. When there were no after school extra-curriculars, it was all hands on deck. With four daughters and a wife, the "girl jobs and boy jobs" business model breaks down in a hurry. There was simply work to be done. Duane was as likely to be found on the business end of a vacuum or with a dish towel over his shoulder as his youngest daughter Leann was milking cows or crawled inside the square-baler with a grease gun.

By the time Leann was a surly, early teen, both Duane and her mother Margie had taken jobs in town and her closest sister was out of college. When she climbed off the bus and into barn clothes, there were three fires to stoke, a herd of beef cows, and a flock of ewes to check. It was a small miracle when a thirty-year-old tractor managed to start against a northern Minnesota winter. When it didn't, the options were to feed by hand or figure out how to use a battery charger.

With fifteen ewes lambing singlets, twins, and triplets by late February, not every one was born head and front legs first. There was no calling Dad on the cell phone, the vet, or the neighbor. When a ewe was in dystocia, you'd find Leann lying face down and shoulder deep searching for a back leg to pull. One Valentine's afternoon she came home to find a lamb lying motionless in the straw. He was nearing room temperature but still breathed, nearly imperceptibly. She stuffed the little lamb under her coat to protect him from the west wind between the barn and the kitchen. She laid him on the bottom rack of the wood-fired cast iron "Daisy", and the cookstove became an incubator. She opened one damper as slight as possible and propped open the door.

Many know Leann the librarian. For those of us who have attended their annual Halloween gatherings, we retain visions of her; graceful and statuesque as Marilyn Monroe or Lady Liberty. To learn that she is adept at setting corner posts square and a gate that swings true, and can hit a nail squarely on the head literally as well as in conversation, requires us to pause. The next time we stop to hold the door for a pretty woman, we realize she may have framed it, hung it, trimmed it, painted it and set the lock. In the case of Leann Lehner, she may have poured the concrete on the sidewalk leading to it.

For her father, Duane Schwandt, growing up in the Great Depression and driving teams of mules in the Korean conflict was little more than a pre-season warm up compared to raising four girls who may have been slow to earn their halos on a farm with two bathrooms: one in the house and one out. When it came to parenting, Duane was self-taught and spot on: discipline when it was deserved, affection when it was needed.

BILL STORK

The day he fell off a barn roof, breaking his elbow, three ribs, his pelvis, and lacerating his liver, he walked fifty yards back to the house. He had a cup of coffee, then drove himself to the hospital. The morning he had to tell Leann the lamb in the oven had passed nearly broke him in two.

Duane Schwandt was defined by productivity, tenacity and multiple permutations, punctuations, and emphasis on his go-to phrase: "Son-of-a-bitch" (ironic for a father of four girls). He accepted help only when it was imposed upon him. By his way of thinking, he wasn't worth a plug nickel unless he was building, fixing, or growing something. To his four daughters, the time when he was not was ultimately impressionable.

He would never allow himself to sit for more than two hours at a time, and only then when he had earned it. When he did, there was a book in his hands, and a cat on his lap, and at his feet.

There were times in her teens when life at 34310 County Highway 4, Frazee, Minnesota, was just short of house arrest. Realization would be a slow burn. By age forty-seven, life on that farm would prove to be salvation.

January 2008, Leann and her husband Kevin were visiting friends and skiing at Lost Trails Mountain, Montana. Halfway between Salt Lake City and Canada, perched at the intersection of the Continental Divide and the Idaho state line. You will find no Californians or Texans. Lost Trails is for locals and friends in the know. The mountain features more than fifty runs over nearly 2,000 acres, but is served by only five lifts. Its base is at 6,400 feet of elevation, and it peaks at nearly 9,000.

As it turns out, 300 inches of powder and two miles of elevation will take a toll on a Minnesota farm-girl librarian. After a few runs, Leann was feeling a bit puny. Owing the sensation to elevation and hydration, she retired to the rental car, reclined the seat and napped as the windshield amplified the afternoon sun.

When in Rome, tour the Vatican. When fortune finds you on a mountain top in Sula, Montana, on a Bluebird Sunny Saturday afternoon, Leann Schwandt is not sitting by the fire and drinking cocoa. After an hour, Kevin woke her from the nap. Raised on a farm where anything short of an open, compound fracture of one or more major long bones was treated with Aspercreme, Bengay or peroxide, she was convinced an epic eructation would set things right. She let fly a "BRAPP!" that would blush Homer Simpson, and they caught a lift to the top.

Buzzing from the thrill of two and a half miles and 1,800 vertical feet of pure powder, Kevin turned to Leann. The chair lift hit their backsides and they lifted off and settled in for the thirty-minute ride to the top. Vibrant and well-spoken by nature, Leann was suddenly gray as the collar of her ski jacket and slurring like the proverbial sailor. Her arms went numb as she struggled to stay coherent. When she leaned toward a sixty-foot fall off the antique lift chair, Kevin thrust his pole to form a gate.

Ski lifts don't do reverse, and the Continental Divide is one of the most pristine places on the planet, largely because it is not cell-served. Urgent and firm, while attempting not to alarm Leann, Kevin began a chain reaction S-O-S. He asked the next occupied chair to summon the ski patrol… pass it on! By the time word made it to the liftie at the summit, the message had morphed into "she's in labor with her first child," but it was nonetheless effective as the ski patrol was waiting at the top.

The Lost Trail Powder Mountain Ski Patrol is an all-volunteer, sixty-two-member team dedicated to the safety of the skiing public and the triage, treatment, and transport of skiers who taco, scorpion, face-plant, or bite it. LTPMSP boasts members who have served thirty years or more on the mountain. Presented with a hyper-extended thumb, they'll have a splint built around your ski pole in time to catch the next lift. A heart attack on the hill will ruin your entire day.

When their chair reached the top, they were met by the mountain ambulance. Leann was draped over Kevin's shoulder like Raggedy Ann. Her gums were pale and heart was racing. Some are EMTs, nurses, and dump truck drivers by day, but on the mountain with their white crosses and red down jackets, LTPMSP are saviors.

BILL STORK

Leann was laid flat in a transport toboggan and wrapped in thermal-foil blankets like a papoose. An oxygen mask was strapped to her face. The strongest of the ski patrollers strapped the yoke of the toboggan to his waist and began the methodical descent to the helipad at the lodge. The mountain was consumed by the gravity of the scene. Like traffic parting for an ambulance on the highway, skiers paused to cross themselves and nod as the armada of ski patrollers tacked their way down the hill. Kevin followed, his entire world reduced to his wife, a wisp of her blonde hair on top of the blanket as her breath fogged the mask.

Their mettle was only beginning to be tested. As the lodge came within view, the helipad was vacant. The silence in the sky was deafening. The nearest cardiologist was ninety-two miles north on I-93 at St. Patrick Hospital in Missoula.

Like a quarterback executing a flawless two-minute touchdown drive, there was not so much as a hesitation. A rented Isuzu Trooper would have to suffice until an ambulance intercept would meet them halfway, in Hamilton. Still in thermal blankets, she was transferred to the passenger seat, barely coherent but nodded her gratitude from behind the O2 mask.

There are times when emotions are not permitted. Before he stepped into the car, Kevin turned to the Lost Trail Ski Patrol, spread his arms wide and partially bowed. The five volunteer professionals returned thumbs up and clenched fists. Kevin's quick thinking and the flawless execution of their training very well may have saved the life of the woman who would come to the rescue of a clueless single dad in need of the perfect Halloween costume.

Her first memory after boarding the lift was twenty-four hours later in Missoula. To find yourself in a hospital bed with an intravenous catheter in your arm and an ECG blipping above your head can happen to anyone. Leann looked up from her pillow to see her right hand being held by her dad. It was then she knew it was serious. Duane Schwandt left his farm to go to church, the feed mill, and the lumber yard. He hadn't been on an airplane since being discharged from the Marines in Korea.

Doctors in Missoula are aces when it comes to broken femurs, clavicles, concussions, and assorted carnage courtesy of the nearby ski hills. Multiple atrial septal defects and a dissected descending coronary artery were "out of their wheelhouse." When her pressures came up, heartrate came down and she cracked her first joke about an impromptu family reunion, doctors determined she was stable enough transfer back home.

Fourteen hundred miles gives a family room to hope. Still, with the best diagnostics in all of medicine, the world class cardiologists at St. Mary's Hospital in Madison looked for viable arteries to bypass or stent. In and out of consciousness, Leann heard the cardiac surgeon speaking to his nurse, "We're going to have to talk to the husband."

She would later relate, "Bill, at that moment I felt the only thing that kept me alive was my will."

She walked out of the hospital a week and seven stents later.

Early this fall, Kevin and Leann adopted two new and ultimately devious kittens. We finished doing their blood tests, vaccines and playing ball with them. The next appointment was running a bit late.

"Leann, when you had your heart attack, do you think growing up on the farm had any impact on the outcome?" I asked.

"Bill," she paused and looked me squarely in the eyes, "it was the difference between life and death. Quitting was not an option."

 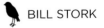

The 'Polar Embrace', or 'Nine Below Zero' Progress Report

Michael Perry is known for his surgical sense of humor. His novel, *Visiting Tom*, made it to number twenty-one on the *New York Times* best seller list. His heartland masterpiece, *Population 485*, has given birth to a culture, and is still going strong. Last year, Mike expounded on a beautiful piece he had written, re-written, edited, and wrestled into place. He stepped back to admire the masterpiece. From the third-person perspective came a realization: there was an element of familiarity to the article. Further research revealed he had written the same piece, word for word, comma for punctuation, three years prior.

Were it not for Mittsy introducing me to the "search document" function in Microsoft Word and the fact that, in sheer volume, I have written roughly the equivalent of an eighth-grade book report (compared to Mike), I would have done the same thing today.

Redirecting, I sat down to expound on the intricacies of the seven-minute nap or my friend Dr. Myron Kebus. Before I could get the first paragraph fleshed out, I realized both were worthy of novels unto themselves. Not to mention it's less than eight hours before Packers vs. Cowboys. There are days for poetry, and there are days for playoff football at Lambeau Field.

Thus, I decided that today would be a fine day to revisit an experiment that began last December, and prove to Mittsy I could write a short article.

You may recall that last winter I made an executive decision: rather than hunker down, hide and complain, I was going to celebrate, embrace and become one with the Polar Vortex. My dad always said, "Don't let your mouth write a check that your [butt] can't cash." Midway through your second pint of Benji's Smoked Chipotle Imperial Porter, it's as easy to say you're gonna buck the winter of 2013-14 into oblivion as "The Packers are going to beat Seattle and go to the Super Bowl."

Well folks, fourteen months in, I'm here to report; mission accomplished and more.

By the first robin's song of 2014, I had six cords of oak split and stacked next to the barn. The dead trees that had fallen on our fence-line in spring had been cleared and burned. There were 200 bales of hay in the mow and another two loads on the ground. It would be just enough to get four quarter horses and Benny the two-ton pasture pet through until first-cutting hay and grazing.

The best part: all the tools you just prop up in a corner because it's too cold to put them where they really belong, and you'll do it when the weather breaks... were put away where they belong. When the weather broke, I went for a bike ride (while waiting for the manure pile to thaw so I could spread it).

The experiment worked better than I could have hoped. To the point there were whole new, I might say earth-shattering, realizations I could have never anticipated.

For my first twenty-one years as a "grown-up," the onset of October meant fresh apples, pumpkin-spice everything, flannel shirts... and doom. Forty-eight degrees F and overcast barely requires gloves, but is the ultimate indicator of what is to come. Under the influence of the polar embrace, I saw epic sunrises diffracted by puddles crunched meeting a chisel-plowed cornfield at the horizon. I saw oak groves, rustling leaves the color of Sheila's auburn hair, piled around her face by her grandma's knitted scarf.

My son was studying on the sunporch. He did not know I could look over his shoulder. In ten random spot checks, he was sending text messages four times, watching ski videos twice and studying American History twice. The *Wisconsin State Journal* recently ran a photograph of people in long lines at the DMV; I found two people with their heads not buried in a smart phone. Every credible new source from the *Wall Street Journal* to *Al Jazeera* have published stories as to how technology is dumbing us down. Fox may have as well. Thanks to instant messaging, navigation, and 4-G, we are rapidly losing our way to plan ahead, commit, communicate, or find our way out of a broom closet.

Try and to stand next to Kevin Griswold's freestall barn last Wednesday morning and send a selfie of you and the cute Jersey. It was twelve below zero with a fifteen mph prevailing northwest wind. Before you could type "me and the girls lol," the device would be frozen solid, your eyes teared up and your texting finger would fall off into the snow bank.

The Polar Vortex (PV) is the ideal antidote for technology.

Find yourself stripped to the waist replacing a left displaced abomasum in the middle of January, your prevailing thought is, "How can I get the greater curvature of the abomasum sutured and my hands back in that hot bucket of water before Steve Yohn opens the overhead door to take the bull calves to Equity?" "Damn, I wonder if she sent a text to tell me she loves and misses me," is on hold until further notice.

Before we wrap up with final thoughts on the Polar Embrace, we take a break from the levity for a warning and acknowledgment: sub-zero temperatures and wind-chills are dangerous, if not life-threatening. I cleared fence and split wood for hours at a time. I was no more than 150 yards from a raging fire and a heated tack room.

There are those who have no home.

Tow truck operators, first responders, firemen, linesmen, plumbers and, of course, farmers often have no such luxuries. They are to be appreciated, respected, and thanked.

Clem "the friendly monster" Mess and I are in lockstep on at least two notions. One is the beauty of old-school country music. The other is the notion that we will not be seen between Halloween and Easter without a stocking hat on our heads, under any circumstances. Fifty years of Cradle Catholicism requires me to confess:

just before sunset on a recent frigid early evening, I found myself twenty-five yards from the mailbox, without a toque.

Sure this was the day the big book deal or Oprah would come through, I consciously overpowered my obligation to brother Clem, and I made a run for it. What happened next I could never have anticipated. I stopped to acknowledge every nerve receptor on my bare skull.

Like the brush of a friend's hand across the shoulder of a widower, it was a sensation I had forgotten, or never known.

It was then I realized I had the power to decide how cold feels on my skin.

I've chosen... peppermint.

Dr. Brodie

In production animal agriculture there is a concept called the Welfare Plateau. It was set forth by a brilliant professor from the University of Illinois named Stanley Curtis. Dr. Curtis was a sizeable man with a photographic memory who moved with great purpose. It was said, and with little exaggeration, if he were to make a sudden stop the first graduate student in his entourage would disappear and may never be seen again. Decorum and respect dictate that we leave the reader to extrapolate Dr. Curtis' anatomic disproportionality.

The Welfare Plateau is not brain surgery. It says that the better feed, water, ventilation, and housing we provide for our animals, the healthier and more productive they will be. One of the parameters that producers and vets monitor closely is timely and efficient reproduction.

It is neither safe nor cost-effective to get the patient to urinate in a cup. With most conceptions being by way of artificial insemination, the bull could be three states away. There's just not that connection for cow and bull to wait the eight minutes for a second line to appear.

Anatomically speaking, the cow's reproductive tract is conveniently accessible per rectum. Veterinarians, technicians, and herd managers have evolved the skill of rectally palpating, or ultrasounding, cows to evaluate their pregnancy state and stage of their cycle. It is routine to sleeve-up and plunge armpit deep into the rectum of a cow. On a harsh winter day, there's no better place for your right arm. When friends come from the big city, I've learned to prep them for what is to come, sometimes.

In 2015, you can earn a pilot's license online, and learn the intricacies of Addison's disease from Google. Palpating cows is an all-in learning experience. Michael Perry's mantra, "Never stand behind a sneezing cow," has never been more relevant. For roughly 3,000 vets who graduated from the U of I between 1954 and 1994, the skill began in the shotgun seat of a Chevy Suburban, halfway between Champaign and Vandalia, Illinois.

In his mid-sixties, Dr. Bruce Brodie bore a striking resemblance to Homer Simpson, if Homer had done a year on Jenny Craig. Substitute the plaid sweater and pipe for a homemade cigarette and a pair of beige Walls coveralls, and he had the demeanor of Bing Crosby on a Christmas special. Just past Effingham, he would clear his throat and look into the rearview mirror to ensure we had shaken off the effects of last night's two dollar pitchers of Budweiser at COD's. After seven years in the classroom, a field trip to the prison with Dr. Brodie was an occasion worthy of pre-celebrating.

He would take the left arm of the passenger and raise it above the dash. Firmly grabbing their wrist he would give a firm shake, "Awright folks, now pretend that Dr. Stork's wrist here is the cow's cervix," he would whisper with the patience of Gandhi. He would rock my hand backwards, demonstrating the move required to bring the reproductive tract into the cow's pelvis. With his index finger between mine, he showed the location of the intercornual ligament and traced my fingers to simulate the uterine horn, finally locating the ovaries at the tip of my fingers.

It wasn't unusual for there to be a token senior on the trip, who would take their turn doing the demo. You could see the squint in the corner of his eye as Dr. Brodie smiled like a proud papa while the student repeated his ritual: line, verse, and pause.

The university had a reciprocal agreement with the Illinois Department of Corrections. In exchange for providing veterinary consultation, we were allowed to bring students into the prison cow herds to learn restraint, treatment, and palpation. To this day, I'm sure they did not consult the cows. Any metaphor drawn from rectally palpating cows at a prison is inferred, incidental, and completely unintentional. The Vandalia prison was a minimum security facil-

BILL STORK

ity, but we were thoroughly searched, and there were strict dress codes that coincided nicely with veterinary fashion. Any sight of skin could incite a riot among 1,300 men who hadn't been to a mall for a decade or more. That worked well. Our blue, green and beige 50-50 cotton Farm and Fleet, short-sleeve coveralls would make Jennifer Lopez as amorphous as an eighth grade boy.

The final demonstration before we would be on our own was priceless. Dr. Brodie would select a Holstein who was both calm and well-fed. He would lube up, deflect her tail and respectfully cone his hand upon entry. He'd curl his fingers and rake any interference onto the barn floor as he stepped away and turned his head. Presented with a whole cow rather than a student's left arm, he would "shake hands with the cervix."

In the time it took him to talk his way around the broad ligaments, horns and ovaries, he would reach into his pockets, presenting a thin white paper from a Zig-Zag wrapper. Selecting just one, he would lay it over her tail head and continue the lecture. As the incarcerated Holstein shifted her weight, he did not so much as stutter as he produced a can of Prince Albert and flipped open the lid. He'd lay a thin line of the aromatic leaf tobacco down the middle of the paper and replace the can to his pocket. Finally, as he reported his findings in the proper lingo: "1.5 CL L, SR," he would pause only to wet two fingers of his free hand and the outside edge of the paper. A finer demonstration of performance art I've yet to see duplicated on any stage. In one smooth motion, he'd roll the cigarette and introduce it to his lips as he pulled from the cow.

Every ten years or so, I'll find my friends Hal Leonard, Edmar Schreiber, or Jon Jorgenson at a continuing education meeting. We never fail to recall Dr. Brodie. When feeling particularly nostalgic, I'm pretty sure I can smell the woody hint of tobacco as I work through a herd check.

Dr. Brodie referenced frequently the work he did in Africa and Egypt, studying the reproduction of the water buffalo that were crucial to survival on that continent.

He never mentioned the four years he fought in World War II.

He also failed to prepare me for Dave Tofte's second cow on the left.

Just as Dr. Brodie had taught me, minus the hand-rolled smoke, I pulled my arm from Dave Tofte's third cow on the left. As I reported the findings on her left and right ovary, there came a thunderous "THWACK!" The sound had a distinct fleshy snap, like the soundtrack of a Clint Eastwood bar scene where he bursts through the swinging saloon doors and lays the guy out with one swift uppercut. In my head there was a distinct hollow percussive tone, like a kid whacking a culvert with a good stout stick.

Exactly my next observation was that I was airborne at a 45-degree angle and on a collision course with the freshly limed barn floor. My next thought; the sound I heard was her foot striking my knee like a line drive to deep left.

I touched down, skidded six inches and bounced. As I curled into the fetal position, I launched a diatribe that would cost me hard time in confession. I may have begged for #2 to kick me in the head as well.

I always seemed to find my way to the Tofte farm around midday. Dave had some right leanings and a taste for talk radio. A temporary loss of consciousness would be the ultimate anesthesia for the knee and I wouldn't have to listen to Rush Limbaugh.

Out of respect for the late Walter Payton and personal pride, I dragged myself to the center post and climbed back to my feet, finishing the last two cows hopping on one leg. Bending my leg to push the clutch was NOT happening. Dave quickly notched a spare two by four to fit the pedal and I hand-shifted down the road.

And so went my introduction to Dave Tofte's second cow on the left.

She was on point at the sound of the V-6 downshifting into the farm drive. If I shouldered my halter and bucket and walked in front of the east bank of stanchions to treat any cow, #2 would smoothly ratchet back and drop her head. Whether my stride was purposeful or tentative the crown of her head would meet my hip at eleven o'clock, just off her left side. Like the ill-fated evening in college, when I was introduced to the cross-member of a lean-to while admiring the rain drip from Becky Bull's brow rather than

BILL STORK

looking for cows and calves, I'd find myself pasted to the fieldstone foundation of the hundred year old hip-roof barn.

Cows have a nearly 300-degree radius of sight, so #2 would never turn her head. Yet, if I were to walk the west side of the barn aisle, she'd stand like a statue made of butter at the Wisconsin State Fair. As repeatable as Rush's lambasting of Clinton: if I were to walk the width of my overshoes on HER side of the aisle... she'd double barrel as quick as a right jab from Sugar Ray Leonard.

In her twelve years on the Tofte farm, that cow endured every ailment eligible to a peri-parturient cow. She had a left displaced abomasum one year, ketosis the next. She retained her placenta, cast her withers, and went lame on all four feet. The rules of her radius never varied; she never granted me an inch of amnesty.

Serendipitous as it may have been, I was on the farm the day she boarded the bus.

Fred Nelson backed down the drive and met the barn door with his trailer gate. Everyone knew about me and #2. I walked her down the aisle and gently prodded as she stepped up. I reached for the gate and she ceremoniously waved her left hoof past the gold stud in my ear. Without a word, I exchanged a smile with Fred and Dave.

I scrubbed my boots and stowed my gear. A phantom shiver shot through my stifle as the V-6 growled from granny low to second gear.

Obituary: Dr. Bruce Brodie

Dr. Brodie (MSU '51), 83, Champaign, Ill., died Dec. 13, 2007. A diplomate of the American College of Theriogenologists, he was professor emeritus of veterinary clinical medicine at the University of Illinois at Urbana-Champaign since 1994. Following graduation, Dr. Brodie practiced in Minneapolis and Delton, Mich. He joined the veterinary faculty at U of I as an instructor in 1954. During his career, Dr. Brodie also taught at the University of Nairobi in Kenya, the University of Alexandria in Egypt, and the University of Zimbabwe. During his sabbatical in Egypt, Dr. Brodie lectured on herd health problems and conducted research on infertility in water buffalo.

He received the 1979 Carl J. Norden-Pfizer Distinguished Teaching Award and the U of I College of Veterinary Medicine's Special Service Award in 1994. Dr. Brodie served in the Army from 1942-1946. His wife, Colleen,; five daughters, and a son survive him. [American Veterinary Medical Association]

BILL STORK

Wide Awake and Feeling Mortal

The second sign came at one of my son's Bantam hockey tournaments, when I found myself engaged in a spirited conversation about blues music and swing dancing with a lovely single lady. As I was looking for a segue to say, "How about a cup of coffee?" Calvin's defensive line-mate crashed the party like a hip-check into the boards.

"Hey, Grandma, thanks for coming to our game," as he gave her a hearty hug.

The first sign was far more emasculating.

Calvin and Paige screamed, "Higher, Daddy!" as I pushed them on the swing set at St. Paul's Elementary school. I was darn near decapitated by my pendulous preschooler as I was distracted by Lee Iacocca's latest temple to the soccer mom rolling slowly down Fremont Street.

"Boy," I thought, "that Champagne-colored Dodge Grand Caravan is a sweet-looking ride."

The very notion that the thought took enough form to earn quotation marks haunts me to this day. For this F-250 and jon boat redneck to have conceived such a notion was a foreshadowing.

There are those who will say that birth anniversaries are just another day. Others require a ticker-tape parade and the University of Wisconsin marching band for turning thirty-two. A card and a cake make everyone feel good. On a sliding scale, I trend toward the former.

"Rock Bottom, population 1…" – Robbie Fulks

Thursday, March 3, 2005. I found myself living in a broken-down rental house on South Main Street, displaced from the home I had planned to retire in. Fortunate, in the sense that I had a roof over my head and two healthy kids. Frustrated to the point that the very next lawyer, family court commissioner, or judge who told me this was a "family redefined" would have found themselves in lateral recumbency. Not so much knocked out, but with their "consciousness redefined."

I was running on vapor when my friend Jen escorted me into the Tyranena Brewing Company. The first sign was a small fleet of Euro SUVs with Illinois plates in the parking lot on a Thursday night. I was met at the door by a cadre of amigos from Chicago, the staff of the clinic, and half the town of Lake Mills. There were the obligatory "Over the Hill" cards, black T-shirts and Rogaine. However, the notion that Doreen would go to the effort to make snacks, dredge up old connections, and reunite the Rhinos was reaffirming to a battered soul.

These days the fence post leans a titch, so that as I swing open the gate to my sixth decade, it drags in the dirt just a bit. Either the milestones are getting heavier or my declining blood testosterone, commensurate muscle loss, and degenerative joint disease just make them feel that way.

Fifty years, by my way of thinking, is closer to the grave than the cradle, but you ain't done yet. By the time I run the next tank of diesel fuel through the work truck, I'll be there.

My friend Gary asked if I had any reflections.

In 1880, the French artist Rodin created his iconic masterpiece *Le Penseur*. The image of deep thought and philosophy has since been that of a giant, naked, muscular guy cast in bronze, sitting on the can with his chin in his hand. Were I captured in a similar pose, the image would be far less flattering. Not to mention, the sitting and thinking would shortly be followed by lying down and Rapid Eye Movement sleep. My Wisconsin 2015 "Thinker" is looking through the windshield of a three-quarter ton Ram, en route to a down cow, on the business end of a snow shovel, or with right arm investigating the many wonders that can be found in a dairy cow's rectum.

BILL STORK

"Doctor my eyes..." – Jackson Brown

I have progressed gradually through stages of nearsightedness and denial. Initially, I could crane my neck and turn my head until I found the sweet spot in my no-line bifocals where I could bring words into focus. Initially, I refused to look over the glasses, and then I tried not to be caught doing it. Now I try to convince myself it looks sophisticated, like Bing Crosby in a sweater vest next to a fireplace.

First, I cursed Wiley and Darby Conley. Their microscopic scribbles in *Non Sequitur* and *Get Fuzzy* look like Rorschach blots to an old guy trying to shovel two bowls of corn flakes by five a.m.

Hoping a confession will set me free, some mornings I will take the glasses off and set them on the counter next to the Tropicana. I've so far resisted the sliding bar in the corner of my screen that enlarges print as big as subtitles at the Highway 18 drive-in. The effects of myopia and astigmatism are inevitable consequences of aging. At age fifty, the images in our rearview mirror should be exactly the right size.

"I wake up in the morning and I know it'll be good, if I stick out my elbows and I don't bump wood." – Bill "The Hammer" Kirchen

The east side of Decatur was appropriately dubbed Dog Patch USA, and we traded goods and services based on a pickup truck economy. It started with a 1970 piss-yellow Chevy half-ton, with a 350 four-barrel and three on the tree. Dad and I hauled firewood for the concrete guy who helped finish our driveway, and a dining room set for the painter who swirled our ceiling.

"Don't jump off the tailgate. Those knees have to last you a lifetime." Dad, the heavy equipment operator, spoke from experience. It's not that I didn't believe him; I just had to figure things out for myself.

I swore I wasn't going to run like an old man. Rubber Tingley overboots, coveralls and all, I can still turn on the afterburners and keep a heifer from getting around a gate. Thing is, I look like a constipated Herman Munster with hip dysplasia en route to an outhouse.

It could have been good fortune, fate, or determination, but right up until the last time my son asked if I'd throw batting practice, I was able to shag his pop-ups all over the infield behind Cambridge Middle School.

One of Jake Untz's cows the size of an aircraft carrier prolapsed her uterus under a stall divider. Jake was flyin' solo as Chuck was shaking hands and making decisions for the Milk Marketing Board in Kansas City. A 200-pound man versus an 1800-pound cow? No challenge. Once I was able to dig a hole in the sand, I had enough strength to wedge myself between the cow's shoulder and the wall, heave her into position and restore her to proper anatomical configuration.

Inspired by the gymnasts in the 2012 Summer Olympics, I attempted a back flip with a half-twist off three bales while loading hay from wagon to trailer. I didn't stick the landing, manifest by blood dripping from a gravel gash on my forehead and two hyperextended wrists. I finished the load with one hand and ratchet-strapped it down. Anxiety overrode my aversion to self-diagnosis; I was two weeks away from a bike trip across Texas. We drove straight to the clinic. Radiographs failed to find a fracture, yet to this day I have cattle-prod-electric pains in my left hand if I curl my left wrist. Typing this story renders my fingers numb. A right-handed palpator of cows, I have yet to miss a herd check.

Two crunchy shoulders have prevented me from military pressing more than 100 pounds for ten years now. Thankfully, there are precious few occasions that require the average dairy vet to lift cattle over his head.

The body has always kept me just out of contention for *People* magazine's "Sexiest Man Alive," but it has yet to fail me. Every now and then, you'll catch me strolling up the hill out back. I come to a complete stop, look skyward and cross myself, mouthing a silent "thank you" to whatever unseen entity may have a part in my functional durability.

"When you comin' home, Dad? I don't know when, we'll get together then yeah, you know we'll have a good time then..." – Harry Chapin

 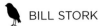 BILL STORK

Parenting at fifty is precarious. I find myself firmly in the grips of P.O.A.D.S. (pubertal offspring acquired dementia syndrome), the disease that affects every parent when their kids are between fifteen and twenty-five. Those so afflicted find themselves capable of writing checks, cooking meals, and fixing things. We can recite our credit card number, expiration date, and secret three-digit number on command. It will be several more years before I know enough to find my way to work without a trail of breadcrumbs. Based on the raised eyebrows, silence and scowls I get every time I speak to my kids, I haven't been cool for years.

For their first fifteen years, you try to bank some cred. The work day was never too long to play catch when you got home. The lumbar was never too creaky for an "uppy" so she could see the clowns in the Town and Country Days parade. My neck never got sore until she asked to get down. *Seinfeld* and *Friends* would wait until *The Giving Tree, Clifford* or *James Herriot's Collection of Children's Stories* had been read for the 135th time for the duration of footy pajamas. There was no bike ride, beer or band that took precedence over being in the stands for every win, loss or draw of their hockey careers. The thought of missing Paige's sprint the length of the rink and diving save that preserved a tie is *the* priceless event straight out of the credit card commercials. As is the malt at Michael's in silence, after the one that got through.

Hypocalcemias, dystocias, lacerations, and obstructions keep gas in the tank and milk in the fridge. You bank goodwill with clients and develop your options with colleagues, so that when the Christmas band concert and awards ceremony come around, you can turn the cell phone *off*. By the time they're making their own decisions, you hope they are able to build the same set of priorities that was demonstrated to you as a kid.

My own understanding took decades.

"Keep the boss-man eating steak and he'll keep you eating hamburger. When the boss goes to eatin' hamburger, you go hungry." – William E. Stork (aka Dad)

Wall Street crashed September 29, 2008. The nation struggled hard for the next four years. Politicians tell us the recession ended in

2012. The single mother with a Bachelor's degree upselling donuts behind the counter at the Kwik Trip has a different story to tell. The technicians at Lake Mills Veterinary Clinic worked harder, longer, and smarter than ever, without hope for a raise in pay, hoping to keep our nostrils out of the water and collections off our doorstep.

The ten o'clock news made daily comparisons to the '80s. What I recall about the '80s is that I never went hungry or cold. My dad was a heavy equipment operator. When highway, hotel, and library construction came to a screeching halt, operator became painter, welder, fixer, and fabricator. When there wasn't steel to be set or a hole to be dug, he carried an F-250 full of grease guns, sockets, and ratchets the size of Fred Flintstone's dinosaur bones. He'd tear something down, build something up or fix it.

As a kid, I can only recall one surly neighbor, and one time Dad being out of work. He was laid off in the morning. Rather than the unemployment office, he went to the Sherwin-Williams. A prideful man, but not to the point he'd risk feeding his family. Eight hours after being laid off, dad was on a twenty-foot extension ladder scraping, priming, and painting Mr. Carter's house.

When there wasn't time to shower before a band concert or honor society induction, Dad would sneak into the back row in chambray work shirt, Levis, and Red Wings.

"Son, there's some things you just won't understand until you have kids of your own," every parent has prognosticated. Well, top dead center, old man. In the meantime you cling to a few words from your daughter that come around less often than a leap year. "Daddy, you just never give up, do you?"

Deep in the grips of my affliction with POADS, it might be a good time to circle back and give the old man his due.

"Bill, which direction isn't important. Just pick one and go like hell." – Stanley Curtis, Ph.D. (mentor to Temple Grandin)

In a story titled "Mary Christmas," I wrote about a farm client and friend: "...the thought that he would have to stand again was the only thing that kept him from falling to the packed snow and gravel and curling up like a fetus." My writing genre is creative nonfiction, which is not to say we don't hide behind a character on occasion.

I consider myself a hard-core commitment guy, but "'til death do us part" was not to be, by ruling of the Jefferson County Family Court. As a parent, I feel like I'm steering a 1975 Oldsmobile Delta 88... from the bumper.

One option is to continue to live in anguish. Twenty years has effectively scrubbed away the patina of insecurity, endocrinology, and expectations that surely factored in what is now a clearly misguided choice.

Equally true is that and every other misstep I've committed have rendered me unequivocally stronger. And, thanks to that lapse, there are two young adults who are without question kind, beautiful, and bound to contribute. Though, on last sighting, the youngest could really use a haircut.

Don Hermann has lost his brother in a truck accident, diabetes took both legs, and his wife left him. The man does not rattle easily. On August 3, 2014, Don did a General Lee into our parking lot, shaken to the core. He pulled up to the clinic, his best friend writhing in pain in the passenger seat of his pickup. Otto had launched from the loading gate of a delivery truck and levered his tibia fibula under the support chain, resulting in a heinous comminuted fracture. I triaged him in the parking lot, sedated and gave him some Torbugesic. I gave Don directions to the Veterinary Emergency Service. Dr. Dana King and her technicians applied four cross pins and external fixators. Twelve weeks later, Otto was chasing chickens and running with the ATV.

We celebrated Otto's return to the starting lineup, but not without a twinge of regret that I do not possess the surgical chops to skip the trip to the referral surgeon.

We spend a lot of time torturing ourselves over what we think we should be. I declare that fifty-years old is the time we allow ourselves to get right with our weaknesses... and to shore up our strengths.

I have a voice, but can't sing like Roy Orbison.

I have two legs, and I'm two years younger than Michael Jordan. I've stood in the tunnel of the United Center close enough to "his airness" to foul him. With MJ in his $1,200 wingtips, and BS in his $150 Red Wings, he's got less than an inch on me. Yet, I couldn't dunk a basketball with a bucket truck.

I have two hands and a DVM behind my name. I'm gonna get good with the idea that I'm not God's gift to a scalpel.

"I don't wanna work, I just want to bang on my drums all day..." – Todd Rundgren.

"You can't beat a man at his own trade," Dad would try to defuse my frustration. Truer words have never been spoken, but I'm working on an algorithm to get right with the acceptable subcontracting of my more marginal skills.

"Son, I'd need a right arm with three elbows and an eyeball on a string," my dad lightly quipped. Curious because not only did he not swear (a habit he admirably broke cold-turkey), but also there was no reference to the engineer who "wouldn't know an 11/16th deep-well socket from a golf tee," whose design required an ASE certified master mechanic and a Yoga guru to accomplish basic maintenance on his 2008 Liberty.

He was referring to the drain plug for the oil pan on his new Jeep. He was seventy-eight years old and it marked the first time in sixty-four years that he didn't change the oil and grease his own vehicle, every 1,500 miles. That, friends, is the tree this apple did not fall far from.

I will stand down from anything that involves automotive electronics, fuel injection, or alignment.

Kim Riege turned our remodeled bathroom into a work of art in six hours for two hundred dollars. I haven't touched a paintbrush since, and I'm at peace with that.

It was rumored that Sam Walton mowed his own grass until the day he died. I'm pretty sure that's what it'll take to get me out of the seat of my Ransome's ZTR, or the John Deere 2520 my dad pre-inherited me. For that matter, I'd be happy to be buried there.

　　　　　　　　　　　　　　　BILL STORK

I still feel an inkling of impotency when I have the folks at Steve's Car and Truck Service change my oil, filters, or bolt a set of mud flaps onto the fender. I'm not yet to the point I can farm out a chunk of my heritage whilst mountain biking, or chasing little white dimpled balls around a manicured cow pasture.

For every skill I realize I do not have, or has eroded, my respect and appreciation of those upon whom I am dependent grows incrementally.

Age fifty seems a most excellent time to get right with who we are. It is a time to give ourselves a break for what we are not, or what we feel we should be.

As a cradle Catholic, you have eight years of CCD classes and confessions ringing in your ears. As a result of being raised in the likeness of Bill and Ann Stork, the notion that you didn't exhaust every ATP to affect your own outcome is not worthy of mention.

When a friend finds themselves in bad way and pulling out, you want yourself to be impenetrable, universally supportive, and brick-shithouse strong. Instead, you allow the notion that your vision of the future is in serious danger of going off the rails to render you selfish. Your girl moved out. Calvin is getting a B in AP physics. Your hip hurts a little. You further torture yourself, like a Mike Tyson sparring partner, because you know Pete. Pete's wife is battling cancer, and his son has mitochondrial storage disease and needs to be fed through a tube. Pete has three herniated disks in his back and drags his left leg.

Just because there are others who have it worse does not preclude us from feeling weak, vulnerable, and depressed. Even if I can't keep my mind there, I find it incredibly liberating to give myself permission to feel the way I do, instead of punishing myself for not feeling the way I think I should.

At the same time, we do not live in a vacuum and *are* obliged to control our outward demeanor and avoid the effects on those we serve, those we lead, those for whom we are an example and those who support us personally and professionally.

"Bill, depression is not a bad thing. It's the pain that motivates you to take action. When it paralyzes you, then it's a problem." – Dr. Ed Fischer

I call myself a cradle Catholic who has backed into Buddhism. On occasion, we have all found ourselves lower than a snake's belly in a wagon rut. We maniacally search like a beagle on scent for an out. Just a word of assurance that a lover can't speak would square us up like Popeye in a spinach patch.

With age comes the experience that there is no quick fix. From the perspective of every emotional state, we have access to a unique set of thoughts that *will* give way to newfound strength. There is no glory in martyrdom; we can allow ourselves to take a break. First, perhaps, for the duration of one song, then maybe an album side. Eventually, a whole concert. Depression is like a trip to the DMV: you're going to be there awhile; see what you can get done while you're waiting for your number to be called.

In time, we come to realize the low times don't last forever, and are followed by compensatory highs. Repeat.

William E. Stork once eloquently stated, "Don't sit on your dead ass and tell me what I'm doing wrong. Show me how to do it right." Don't criticize, demonstrate.

Coaches and mentors offer constructive criticism. Sadly, there are some whose only hope for strength and validation is to take some of yours.

"Ignore the source and the intent, and search for the validity." – William C. Stork

Attila the Hun might say, "You talk with food in your mouth, walk like an oaf, and doubly identify the topic of sentences." If so, then close your mouth, stand up straight, and don't tell me, "I saw Gray, he…"

I'm pretty sure fifty years is a point at which we are supposed to check the score.

While true objectivity is difficult, if not impossible, to achieve, we do know that the denominator is not the dinero. The cars we drive and the label on our lapel matter not. We get closer to knowing if we've earned the oxygen we've consumed when we ask what have we accomplished and whom have we helped.

BILL STORK

Regrettably, there is no ante mortem assessment of our earthly influence. I have been profoundly affected by two Sunday afternoons. In April 1999, I sat wedged between a small army of vagrants and professors at the Oakhurst Presbyterian Church in Decatur, Georgia. In August 2010, I sweltered in a silent line of mourners leading into the Lake Mills Moravian Church that stretched for nearly ten hours. If I can earn a eulogy on par with, if the sum total of the sentiment has a fraction of the substance of, and if mourners have even a few of the same words to say to Paige and Calvin as at the funerals of The Amazing Dick Bass and Brian Krull, I will have achieved some measure of success.

When I talk too long, Sheila drops her chin and half squints her left eye. That translates to: bullet points. If the friends who have helped me celebrate this birthday, my colleagues, clients, kids, and the woman by my side are any sort of indicator... I'm doing okay.

"And when the victor holds your hand up to the great unknown, still you've got to go to sleep alone." – Joe Ely

If we are honest with ourselves, employ every available resource and make the best decision we have the strength for, there can be no room for regret. As Kishan Khemani so concisely pontificated, "Do the right thing."

I'll start by going fishing with Dad, and making a pilgrimage to Atlanta.

The Highland Hillbillies

Somehow it would have been easier if Matt was at least hooked on *All in the Family*, *M*A*S*H*, and *The Jeffersons*.

As a young service professional, I was slower than I should have been to embrace the idea a dairyman can milk cows whenever he darn well pleases. With the late afternoons near his native Jackson, Mississippi, being famously "hotter than a pepper sprout," from roughly three to five p.m. was best spent napping.

A two-hour siesta would be followed by an epic case of inertia. A body at rest stays that way. It would take an hour of *Welcome Back, Kotter* and *Taxi* reruns to get him back in motion. As a result, Matt and Barb didn't get to the barn until most folks were reading bedtime stories to the kids.

When the pager went off about the time the dishes were put away and my couch was calling, nine times out of ten I knew who it would be.

"Evenin'. This is Matt Clampett and I've got an old kayow that's been strainin' to calve, I don't reckon y'all might be in the area and could take a quick look at her..." he would drawl.

One run-on sentence took him longer to speak than to drive to his farm, which is not to say it was close. (Yes, I am fully aware of the hypocrisy.) Instead, I'd use the time to look for something to throw that I didn't need or wouldn't break. All of this was a futile attempt to vent the flash of frustration that would quickly degenerate into a diatribe that inevitably earned me a headshake and a half-dozen Hail Marys from Father Bob at Saturday afternoon confession. To a former Navy chaplain, I was a rank amateur.

 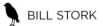 BILL STORK

Matt supposed we'd be in the area and it might only require a *quick* look, an attempt to sugarcoat that only fanned the flame. It also suggested the calf could have been pulled in the middle of the day were it not for his epic insomnia and addiction to late '70s situation comedies.

Nothing on that farm *ever* took place quickly, and "lookin'" was not gonna birth her calf.

By the time I pulled on coveralls and boots and listened to the first half of Fred Eaglesmith's *Paradise Motel* en route, my blood pressure dropped and benevolence returned. Thankfully, Matt's lack of ambition was pervasive. His medical emergencies standardly had a degree of difficulty akin to Greg Louganis doing a cannonball.

Not this time.

He met me at the tailgate as I pulled out my bucket, Nolvasan, lube, and shoulder-length plastic OB sleeves. I left my calf jack for a second trip. In the clinic, if you need to think or consult a colleague, you swab an orifice and excuse yourself to look at it under the microscope. In the country you gotta get something from the truck. Of note to all aspiring country vets, it looks more professional if you bring something back. Not to mention, there was barely room to shuffle sideways through the stacks of newspaper and empty feed bags in the milkhouse.

"Yup, I thought she was gonna calve when I got to the barn this mornin'," he said. Incidentally, most of us here in Wisconsin are eating lunch around "first thing in the morning" on Mississippi Standard Time.

"When we went to the house to take us a rest, she was jest standin' there doin' nothin'," he mumbled like a calf chewing its cud. If ever there were an authority on standing and doing nothing, Matt Clampett would make a county worker look like the Tasmanian Devil on Redbull.

The history that goes, "She started to calve and then stopped" is darn near pathognomonic for a uterine torsion.

(Incidentally, of all the words in my hybrid medical-construction vernacular that spellcheck is mysteriously unaware of, it recognized pathognomonic on the first try. Translated, it means "dead lock cinch.")

Eventually, I would develop a bit of a swagger when it came to correcting uterine torsions and retrieving a live calf. That confidence did not commence until after Francine, the Clampetts' Jersey cross.

Good for more than just reaching the last jar of pickled beets, my arms are long enough to engage a calf's head or hock and my wrists are thin enough to snake through a partially twisted cervix to heave the uterus into more natural anatomy.

On this particular occasion, these long arms were as useful as a trailer hitch on a Toyota Prius. When I pulled on the sleeve and reached through her vulva, I made it to my wrist. My cell-phone suspicion was correct: her cervix was twisted tighter than a loaf of Wonder Bread.

Correcting the torsion vaginally requires being able to get through the cervix, and that was not happening. On other occasions, we would lay the cow down and roll her over, hoping the cow rotates around the twisted calf. That requires an area clear of debris at least three times the dimension of the cow. The Clampetts' dooryard looked like the set of *Green Acres* meets *Sanford and Son*. The nearest piece of naked ground was at the neighbor's farm.

The calf would have to come out the side door.

I was right not to have brought the calf jack. I'd need the surgery kit instead.

What would a surgeon from the human side think of barn surgery? We emptied the two stanchions to the right of our patient and shooed a half-dozen barn cats away. Our scalpels and hemostats were surgically sterile. Two square bales of straw were our standard instrument trays. I once used hay, but a long-necked Holstein thought my surgery table was more appetizing than the silage in the manger in front of her.

LED head lamps were years in the future. Matt's middle son Bobby fetched an orange trouble light with a cage protecting the bulb from under the hood of a Ford LTD in the driveway. On blocks, of course. Edison likely invented the lightbulb in half the time it took Bobby to return. By then, I had clipped and scrubbed the cow's right flank in the shadows. We hung our sixty-watt incandescent rough service surgical light on a nail in the rafters.

A seasoned midwife will famously direct a doting father to go "boil some water and collect as many clean towels as you can find." The farm equivalent is "hold the tail." Just as hot water and towels, it is not a superfluous activity. We try to maintain surgical sterility to every extent possible in a dairy barn. The sensation of a fly on her flank and a switch dangling in the gutter is by definition a violation of sterile prep. Swatted across the face of a veterinary surgeon, it tastes... exactly like you would imagine.

If Matt had strength, it was not his stomach. The notion of impending blood and guts ignited an urgency to start milking. He delegated Barb to be my surgical assistant. Often it takes some gumba to haul a Holstein calf lubed with fetal fluid through a surgery incision. I calculated that Francine's calf would be about the size of a cocker spaniel.

A friend once argued that women can multi-task much better than men. Barb demonstrated in living color.

Her barn slippers scuffed in the lime and cow dung, announcing her arrival before she said a word. The secondhand sweat pants were just snug enough to ensure the pack of Camel cigarettes tucked under the elastic waist band was secure, and just short enough they didn't drag on the barn floor. Her once white V-neck "diego T" provided adequate ventilation on this warm summer evening that surely would have been hindered by any sort of support. Dr. Stork focused on his surgery.

There are considerations to a bovine Cesarean section, beginning with the position of the incision. Too dorsal, and you pull the calf straight up, making it a challenge to close the shrinking uterus. Too ventral, and you risk miles of intestines pouring onto the floor.

Barb paused behind the patient. The motion didn't cease as soon as she stopped walking. I looked high past her left shoulder and emphasized how crucial it would be for her to keep the tail out of my face and Francine's incision. Barb pulled hard on the Camel cigarette wedged between the index and middle finger of her left hand. Gathering gumption for impending battle, she turned and exhaled into the air stream of the barn fan and gulped a dent in the two-liter Mountain Dew bottle. I expected her to find a spot to set down either the cig or the soda, but I'd clearly underestimated the old gal.

Like Dean Martin with a microphone, she transferred the Camel to her right hand to free her left. She hooked the quart of caffeine and sugar with her pinky, and jacked the Jersey's tail.

I prepared to incise. With the transverse process of Francine's back striking me rib high, I positioned my left boot in the gutter and right on her platform—a calculated risk to save my lower back, yet endangering my own ability to procreate in the event the 35cc lidocaine block I used for local anesthesia was not complete.

I pressed the scalpel against the little cow's flank. Like hitting the play button on a cassette player, Barb dumped into a twenty-minute dissertation.

"Hell, I's already eighteen when I went in to have Billy. I didn't figure I'd have no trouble." She paused only to service the cigarette and the Mountain Dew.

"I'd already been pushin' for half a day when that doctor walked in an' asked me if I wanted a shot."

You could feel her pain.

"'Well, Doc,' I said, ' Matt's already been home, milked cows and come back. Good of ya ta take time out of your golf game to give me a hand.'"

I would not have wanted to be that poor obstetrician.

"You can either give me a shot or come close 'nuff so's when I'm feelin' a sharp one comin' on, I kin squeeze yer balls. Thata way, we's all in this together," she bargained.

As fascinating as the intricate details on Billy's birth were, I fought to focus. I had exhausted every option to one-arm roll the calf. I had to calculate the best place to make the incision in Francine's uterus.

I may have missed the old joke about one stitch or two. By the time I was back with Barb, she was breastfeeding Billy.

"That same dern doctor told me that I hadn't ought to be breast-feeding ma own kid." She creased and cursed. In my peripheral vision, she cupped her right hand toward her chest and remembered she hadn't had a drag and gulp for minutes.

"What the hell Doc am I s'posed to do with all this?" She outlined the evidence of her own lactation. "It takes *weeks* to dry up an old cow."

The one thing that went according to plan was the calf was no bigger than expected, and was alone. Anticipating the need, as I fended off the images Barb had made available, she beckoned Bobby. "Hey punkin' head, git yer butt over here and take this calf from Doc soon's he gits it out," she ordered.

The less-than-flattering moniker she routinely hung on her middle son was regrettably accurate. Continuing the comparisons to large fruit, she continued, "Ya' shoulda tried to get that thing out. That boy had a head like a Georgia watermelon the day he was born."

I focused hard on the incision. Still holding the tail and her refreshments, Barb pointed the toes of her slippers wide, bent her knees, and slightly tapped the ashes. She used the glowing tip of the cigarette to trace what I can only hope was a gross exaggeration of the episiotomy incision. "That doc had to cut me from mah crotch to mah armpit," she said, half proud.

Closing a uterine incision the length of the zipper on your Carhartt jacket, while preventing her from depositing her intestines in your lap, is a challenge under the best of conditions. In the absence of the calf, she's trying to involute the organ as you suture, compounding the degree of difficulty. I'm always pleased to have the uterus closed without incident. I had never been so grateful. A three-layer closure of the body wall would take minutes, but it wasn't fast enough. There was the birth of one more Clampett to be narrated.

"When I went to have Bo, I was runnin' the combine," as if that's what everybody does when their third child is about to be born. "I only had ten acres of corn to pick, and it was s'posed t' rain, so's I jest kept goin'," she said flippantly. "Ah reckon we'd a made it t' the hospital on time, but we had to stop at Farstone and get a tar for the grain wagon." She shrugged.

"She just fell out on the truck seat. I didn't figure I'd have no trouble 'tal." Her accent was as thick as the day she left Mississippi. "Now the *same doctor* that told me I should bottle feed Bobby, told me I *had* to breast feed Bo."

Among agriculture-oriented folks, reproduction farm metaphors are free game, as long as everything is going well: "So Pat, heard you got Carrie settled. When is she due to calve?" Everyone laughs.

Matt learned a tough lesson about farm metaphors. "That baby wudn't but two weeks old when I got a hot case of mastitis." Barb winced. She gripped the never-ending cigarette in the corner of her lips, squinted, and shifted the tail to her right hand so she could properly demonstrate the exact sidedness of the infection.

"Matt popped off 'bout rubbin' some liniment on it and givin' me a shot of penicillin in the butt," she said with disgust. "He spent the next three weeks sleepin' on straw bales in the stock trailer." She could not have been more serious.

As I pulled the scalpel blade from the handle and collected my instruments, Francine vigorously licked her new calf. I had done my penance. Barb started the loop again, "Hell, I's already eighteen...," but I felt no obligation to pretend to be polite.

Francine and her calf went on to do well.

I'd give a week's pay for a psychiatrist, priest, or an exorcist to scrub those images from my memory.

The Big Dig

When a concerned client bursts through the door of our veterinary hospital like Kramer on crack, I reach for my inner Steven Wright.

"Doc! It's like he's being attacked from his *rectum*... out."

Four thoughts flashed through my head:

That poor dog.

How can we help?

You couldn't have delivered a more obvious lead line for a story if you'd wrapped it with a bow.

Dr. Ronald Smith

Veterinary medicine is a famously collegial fraternity. This is fortunate. You can graduate from Cornell College of Veterinary Medicine, be certified by a half-dozen different boards, and have two dozen letters after your title. Yet, when your own pet breaks a toenail, you lose your cotton pickin' mind.

It's good to call on these experiences, so when a frantic client lands on your doorstep, you know exactly how *not* to react. Faced with a hyperconcerned client, it is constructive to invert their energy. It allows us to focus on the urgency of the condition, organize the staff, keep other clients from panic, and to minimize the stress of the patient.

It is equally important to communicate concern. Once we had some direction, and the dog relief, we'd surely share a laugh. For now, that had to be stifled.

I chose a square angle to the client, put my pen to the record, and moved to the edge of my stool (pun incidental). We sometimes ask questions to give us time to think: "So, Ken, is this discomfort persistent or intermittent?" I ask, as if it really matters.

Some questions are out of our mouth before we have a chance to think: "How long has this been going on?" I bungle. His dog is acting as if he just lost a jalapeno pepper eating contest with Kishan, Naish, and Sanje. You think he's gonna update his status on Facebook and have a latte, then saunter on down to LMVC? It's a fifteen-minute drive from his place to the clinic; the problem's been going on for eight and a half minutes.

Pruritus Ani (PA) may not be recognized by spell check, but for the staff of most any veterinary clinic, the day is not complete without at least one itchy hinder. Presenting complaints are to the effect of "he's been scooting on the carpet," "he's been licking his back side," or in extreme cases, "he scooted clear down the driveway."

Others require a degree of diplomacy. In a sundress and flip-flops, Michelle sat on the wooden bench. "His breath has just been *horrid*," she says with a most tortuous expression, as the tri-color Jack Russell terrier licks her impeccable complexion.

One would think that in twenty-three years, I would have heard of every conceivable way for a pruritic perineum to present, but alas, it was not the case. To be "attacked from the terminal colon" is either a creative client's way to get moved to the front of the line, or canine discomfort of epic proportions.

Differential diagnoses for PA can include, but are not limited to: urinary tract infections, gastritis, food allergies, and neoplasia. That said, the most implicated anatomy when presented with a history of an itchy butt are the anal sacs.

Experience has taught me that in conversation with clients it's best to enunciate that phrase *very* clearly, refer to them in the singular (anal sac), or to play it ultimately safe and substitute the word "gland" for "sac."

Just a little sinus congestion, background noise, or a poor cell connection can leave a client confused about what exactly you are discussing, and a young vet Badger-red in the face.

Though I have no personal experience, it is horrifying to note that this sensation of which we speak is *not* unique to dogs.

This point was demonstrated in unforgettable fashion to the U of I class of 1992 by Dr. Ronald Smith, DVM, Ph.D.

Dr. Smith apparently has ears like a bat. I would have owed him an apology until the day I passed, were it not for a sense of humor equal to his knowledge of pharmacology and the timing to deliver a nearly surgical touché!

The lecture hall in the University of Illinois — College of Veterinary Medicine Basic Sciences Building circa 1988 had seven rows of desks. The calf-poop brown counter was deep enough for notebooks, coffee cups and big bags of Corn Nuts. The permanent rotating bucket seats were as comfortable as a La-Z-Boy... for the first twelve minutes of each three-hour lecture. The whole apparatus flexed just to the point that, on the off chance a student might doze, his or her head snapped back like a crash test dummy in a K-car.

In the semesters to come, we would learn ambulatory medicine from rock stars like Dr. "Chief" Hornbuckle, surgery from "Cowboy" Dale Nelson, and reproductive physiology from Randy "Bigga is Betta" Ott. It's just not that hard to make collecting semen from a 1,500-pound thoroughbred stallion who ejaculates while airborne, or doing a right flank standing omentopexy on a Holstein dairy cow exciting.

However, it is all for naught without a solid understanding of the basics. Professors like Dr. Smith (clinical pharmacology) were saddled with the onerous task of demonstrating the mechanism by which strategic sugar molecules are bound to the lactone ring of the macrolide antibiotics. As you have certainly deduced by now, it is that structure that allows them to disrupt protein synthesis of some of the more tenacious gram-positive bacteria and stifle an upper respiratory infection or a urinary tract infection.

Slightly built, Dr. Smith was not. One could have easily slipped a three-ring binder filled with a semester's worth of Biochemistry notes into each back pocket of his khaki pants that he cinched securely with a strained black belt, just below his armpits. In the plastic pocket protector he wore on his left breast was an inventory of utensils rivaled only by Office Max. Dr. Smith's lectures were multimedia events, with projectors both overhead and slide. Without looking, he'd whip out the laser pointer and demonstrate the cyclic ester ring that rendered erythromycin exquisitely effective. Then he would deftly switch to the Sharpie, acetate and overhead to specifically demonstrate the inhibition of protein synthesis that could stifle the advance of a stout case of streptococcal pneumonia.

As hard as he tried to make a Hollywood production out of antibiotics, he had to be as glad as we were when the intercom sounded for an eight-minute break.

Drs. Shackelford and Miz simply dropped their heavy heads onto the notes on their desks. Elizabeth Clyde and "Sparks" Revenaugh stood, stretched and assumed yoga poses. Mark Mitchell raided what was left of a twelve-pack of diet Pepsi he had opened that morning. Matt Fraker added twelve ounces of lukewarm coffee to a cup already half-full of Folger's instant crystals.

As we staggered into the hallway, I mumbled to my friend Jon Jorgenson, "He is a nice guy." Which would have been safe, but regrettably I continued, "But that man is dry as a popcorn fart."

Clearly quicker than he appeared, following Jon through the door at that moment was Dr. Smith.

My mind raced to the red pen in his pocket protector and imagined the outright lack of sympathy I had just earned on the day we were tested on this material. I glanced quickly to the corners of his eyes, the edge of his mouth, and his brow. I wasn't much for suspense and needed to know how many percentage points I had just cost myself.

The man did not flinch.

Six minutes later we returned to our plastic seats. Only two hours left. I thought I was safe from repercussions from my earlier remark.

We thought nothing of it as Dr. Smith seemed to fast-track through the clinical relevance of the -mycins. Without so much as an

BILL STORK

inhale, he launched right off into the -cyclines.

Not one of us minded as he flashed rapidly through slides demonstrating the four hydrocarbon rings that gave tetracycline its name and function, but when he arrived at precautions and side-effects, he dropped right back down to granny-low.

Most of us were aware that tetracyclines administered to young animals could result in brown-stained enamel teeth. A few may have known that doxycycline could cause esophageal strictures in cats if not properly irrigated with water or lubricated with butter.

None of us were aware of the potential side effects of tetracycline antibiotics in humans.

Dr. Smith featured a slide mentioning the tiny percentage of *human* patients who could experience a reflex intestinal dysbiosis as a result of the antibiotics. This is an overgrowth of bacteria in the duodenum and jejunum that, in the presence of adequate carbohydrates for growth medium, could lead in some cases to an inflammatory bowel.

Most professors think nothing of self-deprecation for the sake of education. Dr. Smith described a summer he spent at Rocky Mountain Biological Research Center in Gothic, Colorado. He came away with an album filled with pictures of Maroon Belles at sunrise, and the alpenglow of sunset over high-mountain lakes. He also returned with a debilitating case of Rocky Mountain spotted fever.

With his history of travel to the mountains, an alert physician at University Health put him on 100mg of tetracycline every twelve hours, and promised an excellent prognosis for a full recovery. Within seventy-two hours, the aches and fever began to subside, in precise coincidence with the onset of one of less frequently experienced side effects of the drug in humans.

"Dr. Stork," he raised an eyebrow at me, "do you care to hypothesize as to the consequences of an intense case of inflammatory bowel, should it proceed ante grade in the tract?"

Rather than wait for me to stammer an answer, he began to walk slowly across the stage, then picked up speed rapidly. By the time he made it to center stage he was fast-walking like the Saturday morning tribe of soccer moms on the North Shore of Chicago.

Recreating what had to be a harrowing experience for a self-conscious, introverted undergraduate, he mimicked ducking behind a tree, then reached around and buried his hand between the pockets of his khaki pants. Curling his fingertips, he dug and scratched furiously.

Stepping back to the podium, he winked and pointed in my direction. With a perfect poker face, he waited as eighty veterinary students struggled to regain composure.

As you can imagine, an exaggerated case of lower GI inflammatory bowel becomes, by definition, an obligatory case of *pruritus ani*... of epic proportions.

BILL STORK

Dear Sarah

From an online review:

Not at all in Herriot's Shadow

This book was such a colossal disappointment that I didn't even finish it. The author doesn't write much about animals at all, and never with the grace and self-deprecating humility of James Herriot. It's a didactic and overtly Christian tome. Reading it is like being stuck in a discussion with an overly prideful person who can't get over the "good 'ole days." Sarah K.

Sarah, I've been anxiously awaiting your input. In the nearly seven years since I've put pen to paper and Mittsy has labored to edit these chapters into form, I've learned a lot.

We've been reviewed by many in overwhelmingly kind fashion.

"Dr. Bill, thank you so much for writing this book and helping restore my faith in good people," wrote our good friend Lisa.

"Bill, your book is better than I thought it would be; I never realized what I was missing," from Janet Peterson.

The praise is very gratifying; I am thankful that it came first. Kind words spoken as the first few stories were printed from the likes of Don Grant ("Doc, I love the humanity of your stories") were like hot dog bites to a lab pup learning to sit. They provided the reinforcement I needed to get comfortable putting myself out there.

Not every evaluation was wholesale kind.

"I liked the book, Bill, but sometimes I just didn't hear your voice coming through," Mike Kelly offered over a pint on a Thursday night.

"Doc, you introduce us to all these fascinating people, then you move on. I would really like to see you develop your characters more completely," offered Carl Zinser in the foyer of the Watertown Farm and Fleet.

The pragmatist in me always knew you were out there. I am sure some detractors simply put it down, recycled it, or used it for kindling on a cold day, either too polite or lacking the energy to take the time to write a review. I would have preferred to smash my thumb with a ball-peen hammer than read your words, but I planned to internalize the critique, and get better.

What follows is my response to your well-thought comments.

Not at all in Herriot's Shadow

Simply put, I chose this title as Dr. Wight was a veterinarian in a small town in England; Dr. Stork is a vet in a small town in Wisconsin. (I reckon it's too late to choose a pen name.) I truly regret your disappointment if you spent your hard-earned money expecting a 2014 edition of *All Creatures Great and Small*. I read Herriot in eighth grade, and not a word since. I call the series "the books that cost my construction-working dad an eternity of overtime and $150,000." I don't recall a thing about how to treat animals, if he even mentioned it. The impression that has endured for nearly forty years is the reverential feel. The kinship he shared with his herds, patients, and friends, and the nobility with which he and local icons like Dr. Leland Allenstein represented himself, his family, and our profession is well worth emulating.

The author doesn't write much about animals at all

Sarah, we let you down there. By way of full disclosure, we sent the original document to the publisher arranged roughly chronologically. We thought they would surely move Cooder, Sallie, or Buck to the front of the line in order to engage the animal lovers. In hot pursuit of a deadline, that did not happen. By page 108, I made it out of veterinary school, and still had enough hair to justify going to a barber to get it cut flat on top. At that point came needy cats like Pumpkin, and comical dogs like Remmi, Cooder, and Token.

In a sense, I am more in Herriot's shadow than you may know, and not in a flattering fashion. Dr. Herriot was a huge soccer fan. He wrote extensively about sports and everything *but* animals. For twenty years his words fell on deaf ears, and those who were listening were anything but kind. Maybe I should follow his lead and send a few copies to England. When he finally sat down to write animal stories, they went nowhere in his hometown. It wasn't until a reporter for the *New York Times* was moved by his work that he finally took off. Then again, he didn't have Facebook.

...and never with the grace and self-deprecating humility of James Herriot

"Cat's in the Cradle" was a piece written for Father's Day. As you may have read, my dad was never too tired to play catch with his son, even after climbing crane booms 250 feet in the air with a sixteen-pound sledgehammer. He ran any machine from a Bobcat skid loader to a 500-ton tower crane with the precision of a surgeon's scalpel. There are libraries, gymnasiums, swimming pools, roads, bridges, and a nuclear power plant that will stand for a century as monuments to his productivity. He defined "in good times and in bad, in sickness and in health" through a decade of dementia until death did finally part he and my mother.

He refers to himself as "a dumb-ass construction worker."

Carl Zinser could be anywhere from 65 to 110 years old. He lives in the farmhouse he was born to. Carl farms eighty acres and raises twenty or so calves a year. He wears secondhand clothes, Velcro shoes, and gloves that don't match. He could keep my friend Neal the dentist busy for the rest of his career. He also speaks with impeccable grammar, quotes freely from the thousands of books in his library and knows the stock market like Warren Buffett. He has contributed valuable input to these stories.

Carl begins every sentence with, "Now you have to realize this is coming from a dumb old farmer..."

As for the self-deprecation that you are missing Sarah, I respond twice.

The first being, I have long felt that the enormous majority of human behavior is managing our insecurities. As optimal as my upbringing may have been, "just a dumb old construction worker" ringing in my ears may have imparted the notion that everyone else is smarter or better than me. A deficiency of self-deprecation may be a conscious effort to separate myself a bit from one thread of my bringin' up.

Aside from that, I've no choice but to own my own shortcomings.

Secondly, on the topic of self-deprecation deficiency, I refer you to "Pumpkin" and "Under Pressure."

As for the grace of Dr. Herriot... I can only aspire.

It's a didactic and overtly Christian tome

As for the didactic tone you felt, I admire that you exercised your prerogative. If you aren't getting graded on it and if you aren't pickin' up what I'm puttin' down, then walk away and write a review.

With regard to the overt Christianity, I was concerned. Though I am a Christian and person of faith, I have *no* less respect for those who are otherwise aligned. My editor was raised in Tennessee as a Baptist. As an adult, she came to develop beliefs that were not consistent with the teaching of John Smyth. In that transition, she developed an extremely sensitive gag reflex for things perceived as righteous or religious. She became my "sermon beacon." Your threshold is more sensitive than ours and I apologize.

I am a cradle Catholic who's morphed into the cafeteria variety, and backed into aspects of Buddhism (see "I think I Can"). More than denominational, I'm a person of very simple faith. Whether I'm delivering a calf or negotiating with my son, I require that I do the absolute best I can. If I have first prepared, and then spent every single ATP physically and mentally, I can accept the outcome.

Those who do not embrace the existence of a deity would argue that's simply an exercise in trusting oneself. To which I answer, "Yup, sounds good to me."

My faith accounts for the appearance of Mary at the exact moment a good man was about to end his life, Sallie barking at a stove, and Bambi. I leave others to interpret as they wish.

BILL STORK

It is also true that many people I admire, if not aspire to, are void of those beliefs. In a story that has been written since IHS was released called "Family Tradition," a very good friend found herself precariously balanced on the thin edge between life and death. She credits her survival to having grown up on the farm... and her will. I silently add an element of divine intervention. Leann has no such belief. It's only a conundrum if you let it be.

Reading it is like being stuck in a discussion with an overly prideful person who can't get over the "good 'ole days"

Sarah, up to this point, I'm on board with you. But on this one, you've got my hackles up a bit. At no point in 264 pages of *In Herriot's Shadow* or fifty years of my life have I felt an inkling of personal superiority. I've saved my superlatives for the people I've consciously borrowed pieces of.

There are times I can be moved to tears by memories of The Amazing Dick Bass; I am grateful for every minute I spent on a stool at a donut counter with him. It is not humanly possible to be *overly* proud to have been raised by my parents and to know Kishan Khemani, Scott Clewis, Gary Edmonds, Jay and Joy Lou Walker, Jim or Roger Kassube, Jean Jensen, The Vergenz, Mittsy Voiles, John Humphries, DonMary Grant, Clem Mess, Vernon Strasburg, Lyle Wallace, Chris Roedl, The Haacks, The Wollins, the Healys...

"Stuck in the good 'ole days" could imply a failure to embrace technology, to which I answer: I'm writing what you read on my laptop computer and next to my bed I have a 4G tablet to keep up with breaking news and to update the status on my three Facebook pages. In my pocket at all times is an Android-equipped smart phone. On it I have libraries full of high-res photos of excretions, secretions, and abnormal stool from my patients. I have video sent at all hours by concerned clients whose dogs are reverse sneezing or experiencing limbic seizures, and whose cats are looking for love.

My son Calvin once told me, "Dad, that's old school."

I will not pirate the music of a musician who's ever known my name, played for a crowd of people smaller than my immediate family, or shaken my hand.

I drive across town to buy a head of lettuce from the grocer who sponsored my son's soccer team, and a six-pack from the family who brings their cats to our clinic.

I will pay ten more dollars to buy a cordless Milwaukee Sawzall from Dave at the Cambridge Ace Hardware. He's just down the road and stayed open late and dropped off the rinse and vac when Token was a pup.

I write of hard work, faith, family, and accountability.

So, Sarah, if that constitutes being stuck in the past... guilty as charged.

BILL STORK

Oh, Lord, It's Hard to Be Humble (aka Dear Mac Davis)

Mac Davis didn't know many farmers.

I swore I wouldn't become one of those old guys. If I did, I wasn't going to whine about it.

I'm 0 for 2.

The amount of effort required to achieve vertical is in direct proportion to minutes spent sitting and who's watching. Sleeping on my left side or embracing for long periods of time renders my left hand paretic. For the past fifteen years, from late September through April, my index finger turns white and throbs. Dave Strasburg's Holstein #1226 had spent more time at the top of the Dairy Herd Improvement Association than the Beatles on Casey Kasem's American Top 40 when she displaced her abomasum. Her productivity was matched only by her spirit. She was not in the least impressed by a combo line-paravertebral block 60cc of lidocaine, a half cc of Rompun, and Dave's best tail hold. We made our skin incision without incident, but when my scalpel found a superficial epigastric nerve the lidocaine had not, she delivered a roundhouse with her right rear quicker than Dr. Dave Rosen in a bar fight. The deep bruise on my quadriceps has long since healed, but as she hiked, I plunged the scalpel deep into my finger. I felt the fire, and the glove fill with blood. I'm still waiting for the medial metacarpal nerve to regenerate.

When counting blessings, I don't have to look far. The woman I've spent much of the last six years with is beautiful beyond what I could ever hope. She is compassionate, frugal, and accountable, attributes I fondly recall while sweating and scrambling to put up hay in the north mow of the barn with her nephew.

Sheila does not shop for things she does not actually need, cowboy boots and jeans notwithstanding. I've never had to search for her car in the parking lot of a bar. If she's gone missing, she's in the barn, taking care of one of her eleven horses.

Respectful of our time, she's looking to get done. You peer through the dust and sweat on your glasses for an opportunity to grab a bale without having your spine compressed. Occasionally there will be a sliver of daylight between the next two bales.

There is science, art, and etiquette to putting up hay. You pick a pace you can maintain until the wagons are empty, walk 'em, don't throw 'em, and alternate hands. You start every new row from the outside and look to locate rogue spaces that can be filled with an edgewise bale. The hay will be loaded out when there's a lot less daylight. When you sell a load to the neighbor with goats, and his boot doesn't fall through, he may not say a word, but he'll loan you his post-hole auger without having to ask.

The most important rule, no matter how many are on the wagon and how few are in the mow: the minute the last bale falls, you settle your breath like you've been reading a book and sipping tea. You scramble down to the mouth of the mow and ask, "Y'all need help bringing the next load around?"

We were a dozen bales down when Bryce bent over to grab his jeans like timeout in double overtime. "Either we're really out of shape, or she's out of her mind."

I assured him he was dead-on in at least one respect, but a mound of loose hay on the floor of the mow had left a three-foot wave in the corner.

"No way, Bryce, it's all these broken bales," I gasped.

"I don't give a damn, let's just let 'em drop. She won't know until this winter." He knew better.

I can only be grateful there were no witnesses to the pre-"Vitamin

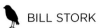 BILL STORK

I" (ibuprofen, extra-strength) segment of Monday morning. I can only hope that double amputee Don Hermann gets out of bed with more grace. I wasn't obligated to achieve full vertical, so I didn't push it. Proving that physics touches our lives on a daily basis, I discovered that underwear can be installed with the contralateral hand on the counter, compensating for a sore right hip.

Some time ago, as I turned north off Navan and onto West road en route to the Tim and Lisa Claas farm, the ditches were in full glory. There were a precious few phlox making an encore, the dusty, fragile blue flower decorating the barbed-wire spine of the chicory as it flourished in the gravel on the shoulder. Thankfully, Tim milks late. The lethargic day lilies had finally yawned to life, dominating the ditches. The garlic mustard weed lent an aroma accentuating fresh cut hay, and obliterated all but a few surviving red columbine.

As if I didn't know the way, the roadside came alive with a swirling gauntlet of yellow finches, bluebirds and chickadees to lead my way.

If attitude is everything, perspective is the rest.

Had Michael Perry, Fred Eaglesmith, and Glenn Fuller been in the car with me, Fred would have written a song, Mike would have written a story, and Glenn would have photographed and then drawn the image.

It was on that visit Tim and I gossiped at the tailgate, after we had pregnancy-checked his cows. I noticed a mountain of chaff at the base of his hay elevator and six empty racks.

Attempting some semblance of solidarity, I shared my Saturday in the mow at the Barnes farm. "How much did you put up?" I asked him.

"Between Thursday and Sunday I put up 4,400 bales," making our 250 seem like doing dishes for a tea party. Searching for redemption I asked, "Who'd you get for help?"

"Brian helped for a while on Saturday." He shrugged lightly. I'd need the Wisconsin National Guard.

Hastily changing the subject to the ten inches of rain my dad got down in central Illinois, I fished for the two bottles of Lutalyse, oxytocin and GnRH he had requested.

Tim shuffled back to the barn, his right Tingley rubber scuffing in the gravel, two sizes larger to accommodate the walking cast.

He raised his head rather than wave, the medicines cradled between his hand, his chest, and his stump.

BILL STORK

You Can't Handle the Truth

"Just outta curiosity, what the hell qualifies this as a trail?" gasps Mike, through lips pursed tightly to drive every molecule of oxygen above 10,000 feet across his alveoli to his increasingly hypoxic blood. Framed by a snow-white, Hulk Hogan Fu Man Chu, you're ten times more likely to hear a laugh like the back room of a bear cave come across the electrician's lips than anything resembling a complaint.

Thursday, August 6th, had begun as most on a Lizard Head Cycling trip. The sun had begun to glow. Travis Tucker had two blue granite kettles of Ophir Spring Water to a rolling boil long before the sun had crept over Teocali Peak to melt the frost off tent flies.

Like reveille at boot camp, "Coffee!" bellowed through cupped hands set in motion a relay past the twin Aspens and just over the ridge to a World War II ammunition box with a white acrylic lid. The relay baton is a shrinking roll of Charmin in a plastic bag. The Groover is so called for the impression it made on campers before the acrylic accoutrement. It is strategically placed 200 feet above Brush Creek, raging with runoff from April snows and June monsoons. It ain't no bidet at the Ritz, but everyone goes home with a series of pictures labeled "Views from the Groover."

Thirty minutes later, the twelve-inch cast iron Mountain Microwave sizzling over the third burner of the Coleman Pro yielded two dozen eggs, peppers, potatoes, onions, and seven pounds of coffee-rubbed beef brisket. I presented my tin camp plate with two whole wheat bagels slathered in honey butter and buried 'em with two shovels of rocket fuel. A bowl of Special-K and a glass of skim wouldn't get you to the trailhead today. For dessert, there was fresh fruit, yogurt and granola.

The real men of the mountains plowed through bowls of Steel Cut Oats with overhand grips on soup spoons the size of gravy ladles.

John, Travis, and Less-lie recovered the kitchen. In anticipation of the impact of the trail, many of us titrated bottles of electrolytes, threw down handfuls of Vitamin-I (ibuprofen) and strategically slathered Chamois Butt'r. Terri gathered our attention by demonstrating how to distinguish a housewife from a prostitute, using a banana as a prop. We all crossed our hands and bowed our heads as she seamlessly segued into a non-denominational request to be safely delivered back to camp.

Before he rolls out the more conservative (slower) riders, John Humphries gathers his crew around a laminated trail map of Crested Butte. With a broken stick as a laser pointer, he traces a high-lighted series of trails that cumulatively look more like Ferdinand Hayden's original circumnavigation of the Elk Mountain Wilderness looking for gold in the late 1800s.

The rookies laugh as the guide issues the first disclaimer of the week: "How do you tell when a guide is lying? His lips are moving."

For the first five years I laughed like it was the first time. Each of the ten years since, I've developed a growing measure of disdain for the lighthearted self-deprecation. Mountain guides are among the hardest working, most skilled and dedicated professionals I've ever known.

It starts with how they describe their office. With the reverence of a farmer in his field, they enunciate every syllable and sound when they refer to the Elk, the Maroon Belles or the LaSalle "Moun-tens."

"We'll climb up Brush Creek Road to just past the outlet for the Teocalli Trail." He looks around for nods of acknowledgement from the previous day. "Just past, and on the opposite side of the road could be a sign for Cement or Marble Creek Trail," he speculated. "Once you find that, go through a gate and take a left. There you'll start a climb at the base of the 405 trail." He could not guarantee a marker.

BILL STORK

Clearly uneasy at the notion of sending a couple Californians and a flatlander off into the mountains ("If you are ahead of the guide, you are no longer on a guided trip"), John called a Hansel and Gretel. "Find three sticks and make an arrow in the grass next to the trail."

I leaned in close to look over my bifocals. The contour lines connoting elevation gain merge imperceptibly to black. I thought to myself, though I spoke not a word, "If you ain't hikin', you ain't bikin'" will be fully enforced until further notice.

Expedition mountain biking is like a week-long equation; the trail itself being a four-dimensional, twenty-five-mile puzzle. Every ATP is to be carefully budgeted like last week's paycheck. You sight down the trail to see a hard pitch with off-camber roots and a "grave yard." You negotiate with your legs, lungs, and mind. Go hard early in the day, and risk blowing up after dinner.

Mike and Phil opt to push the big hills on Brush Creek Road. I resolve to spin in granny low. I refuse to give up my seat until the single-track. We are blessed with a sign that marks the Perkins Trail. Mr. or Ms. Perkins is either one heck of a bike rider, or a practicing masochist with a sick sense of humor. In twenty-five yards, the trail turns straight south, pitches 27 percent and disappears into the aspens. Grooved deeply by a decade of 250cc moto-tillers, we are a line of three marching at a sub-glacial pace, pushing our $3,000, full-suspension machines up the first of the hike-a-bikes. In a quarter mile, the trail mellows nicely and we roll through a deciduous forest.

Through a cattle gate and pasture, we encounter another bifurcation and call a map session. Clearly our trail continues the contour, but to ensure we don't do a three-man Christopher McCandless, we gather wind-fallen aspen branches and form another arrow in the grass. As the single track gives way to an ATV trail, the trees part over a mountain meadow shared by bike riders, hikers, and a herd of Red Angus heifers. We pause at a trail sign to confirm our orientation. As a rider in full armor idles up the trail, the sanctity is broken by a war whoop and pace line led by John. Tim, Mr. Stu, B-Rob, and G-Rob ride up our backside.

When a guide's lips move, truth may be optional, but is worthy of note: he is also responsible for hemostasis, stabilization, and evacuation of fallen riders. (Not to mention, injured or hospitalized riders do not famously tip well.)

"Now that we're all warmed up," he understates, "there is a section ahead Fred calls The Rock Garden." Fred has lived in Crested Butte for twenty years; his perspective on the relative navigability and potential perils of a trail is not to be ignored. This Rock Garden will not be some backyard art piece built with a Bobcat and a landscape architect in a high-dollar second home suburb.

A guide by nature, a teacher by nurture, John begins a mountain meadow physics lecture on momentum, leverage, torque, and trajectory that will preserve our tires, rims, and shins.

Nearby, the herd bull chewed his cud. Back home, I've been escorted under a barbed-wire fence and vaulted a gate just a few strides ahead of a couple Holstein bulls. This guy rose lazily and stretched. He sniffed the breeze and flared his nostrils at the unmistakable scent of an LH surge. He searched for a strand of clear mucus. Clearly his eighteen young heifers looked, and likely smelled, better than a troop of skinny, sweaty yahoos on bikes. There was plenty of mountainside for all of us. Passing on his superior genetics was clearly a greater priority.

John answered the question before it was asked. "There will be some climbing after the garden. We'll do another re-group at the top and have the first sandwich, before a big descent." His measured enthusiasm for the downhill and emphasis on "first" sandwich was foreshadowing.

Proving that a body in motion will stay that way, and one who looks at the boulder he seeks to avoid, does not; I careened off a boulder the size of a VW Beetle. In doing so becoming at one with the mountain and donating an ample sample of my DNA. From the six-inch excoriation trickled a steady stream of serum into my Smart Wool socks.

Mountains are not to be conquered so much as revered, and left with as little trace of your presence as possible.

BILL STORK

Having achieved our first summit, Frank spent half of his word count for the entire week. "So, how much of the day's climbing have we done so far?" Useful information as we toggle between attempting to budget our waning resilience versus staging an injury and playing our three dollar Colorado Evacuation Cards.

"We did not invent the truth, we just manage it," goes the old lawyer joke. Surely plagiarized from a guide.

One of the subtly spoken goals of John and Lizard Head is to wean us off our GPSs and watches, and measure our moments in units of suffering and summits rather than watts and miles. By Thursday, we all knew better than to expect a quantitative answer. In order to prepare us for the rigors of the trail ahead, without inciting a mutiny, he reached for a metaphor from the world of combat sports.

"Well, it's a bit like a fight with Mike Tyson. You've just made it through the first round," as if to be encouraging. "He tried to take you out early with punishing blows to the head and body." He continued the happy news, "After a spectacular downhill, there will be a mile of climbing on a 'road.'"

There will be climbing. There will always be climbing. On a Jeep trail we should be able to earn some elevation with the only obstruction being a 25 percent incline.

Or so we hoped.

Back to the battle with the bipolar heavy weight champ. "You will think he's giving you a break, and then he'll try and take you out with a flurry of punches."

We sat 2,000 vertical feet above the valley floor. The heartiest whole-grain ham and cheese doesn't fare too well in a backpack. We sat plowing our sandwich balls and taking long hard pulls from the bite valves of our CamelBaks. West wind delivered the flatulent braap of a Jake brake from a semi that looked the size of a Smart Car, slowing a delivery into Crested Butte. Through a slit in the aspens, we could catch the reflection of Highway 135, the first evidence of civilization in seventy-two hours.

My son Calvin calls the national car of Colorado "Rainbow Racers." Nearly every Subaru into and out of town is drafted by four bikes on the receiver racks. 3-Rivers Paddle Shop cinch straps secure kayaks and SUPs; loose ends dangle in the breeze. Highway 135 is the only route in, and there isn't a paved road out of Crested Butte, Colorado. There are no water parks or duck-boat rides. The magic show at night is the Milky Way, undiluted and unobscured by light leaks and air pollution. The closest thing to McDonald's, Starbucks, and a La Quinta is The Last Steep, Camp 4, and The Old Town Inn.

It is no longer the best kept secret in the Mountain West, but there can be nothing wrong with babies and backpacks. From grandpa to grandson, three generations in hip waders stand downstream. They draw sine waves above their heads in DayGlo line and mono-filament leaders with split bamboo fly rods. The Gothic River yields rainbow and brook trout for a hearty lunch and images of a life-time. The rest would be gently cradled and returned to the water to swim another day.

Leash laws are as follows: "Please keep your dog within reasonable vocal distance; if he eliminates on the trail, kindly kick it to the side."

The descent from 409 trailhead would make 4k-Ultra High Defini-tion TV like a mimeograph of a Monet. Ahead of me, G-Rob parted fields of helmet-high wildflowers like the Harvard heavyweight skull on the Thames. Silently the vegetation falls shut behind him. The soon-to-be father on his last kitchen pass disappears down a trail by blind faith and braille. Fighting to ensure I was looking two lengths ahead, my driver's side peripheral view was full fields of corn lilies, mountain lupine, and monument flowers, fertilized by historic spring snows and summer monsoons. Their edges, serrated like a Ginsu, were like Grandma's cheese grater on my newly ex-posed sub-cutis. The neoprene leg warmers in my backpack would serve nicely as an Ace bandage. Rather than break my flow, I opted to embrace the sensation and employ the cowboy adage: HDFU (paraphrased and translated: "get tough").

The trail hugged the cliff like the window ledge in the movies. The passenger side view dropped a thousand feet to Slate Creek, winding like a kitten's ribbon in the valley floor.

 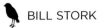 BILL STORK

Miles of trail and a thousand feet of elevation gained in hours, step-by-step and in granny low evaporate like ninety seconds on a roller coaster. When John appears again he's pointing up the road, while adjusting the travel on a hydraulic disk brake. "And here begins the death mar..." he catches himself, "I mean, the second climb."

Hypoxia had eroded my loyalty when Travis ground to a halt, having over-powered his drive train and stripped his hub. A thought came. If I were to turn down this so-called road, I'd eventually be a part of the paved parade heading into CB. Travis and I could coast into town. We could walk up Elk Avenue and have a beer at The Steep and an Americano at Camp 4. We could poach a piece of binder twine from a construction site, and I could tow Travis up Brush Creek Road into camp. A calculated risk, but surely less painful than the next few rounds with Tyson. I had lost my mojo and mindset to tempt fate and double back through the Rock Garden, this time as a downhill.

John's "road" was more painful than two days in divorce court. Folks always want to know, "How many miles?" Trying hard to separate mind from body, I called on Kristofferson, "Freedom's just another word for nothin' left to lose," and waited for Tyson's next attack.

Which took one more chorus, "I'd trade all my tomorrows for a single yesterday."

In fifteen years of travel with John, we've hiked over the Continental Divide, been chased off the Indian Ridge by a wrath of God electrical monsoon, and endured a campsite known by locals as The Vortex.

I thought I'd seen it all.

The "road" came to an unmistakable end and funneled us to the foot of what more resembled an avalanche chute or climbing camp for a Navy SEALs program. The nine men ahead of me labored in silence. B-Rob looked for the next footfall and a line to push his bike; he found neither. Mike struggled to find the shoulder technique. G-Rob, with quads like John Kuhn and two years short of the big 3-0, stood bolt upright in utter disbelief.

A guide finds himself accruing and spending cred, going from boom-time to belly up and back again between breakfast and dinner, every day. Sensing his account was about to be overdrawn, John kept it simple. "Pick a number," he said, sounding like a card-trick magician at a ski lodge. "Take five steps, then five breaths," as if we could find a place to put our feet without tumbling back to Highway 135. "Then repeat." He assured us we would reach the top.

Once the 405 turned to what could be classified as a trail, we collapsed like survivors in a plane crash. Mr. Stu filtered stream water, Tim cooled his bottles in the stream, and John found a hole deep enough to immerse his entire head. Frank and Phil squeezed the last of their sandwich balls from the Ziplocs.

We were rewarded with a lush, cool pine forest and a trail that crossed the stream and contoured for an easy mile or so. When the trail pitched hard to a cobalt blue sky, we sensed that Double Top was in range.

"Pick up your head, men. It is said the aspens have eyes." He begged us not to miss the majesty. Indeed the gnarled, darkened bark resembled wise old men. The trunks leaned nearly imperceptibly as the tops reached to the sky. John pointed and we stopped to pick wild mountain strawberries from the low bushes that lined the trail.

With legs and lungs on fire, the trail on my passenger side dropped off into infinity. I bought the high side of the last rock formation and cleaned the 401. The trail leveled into a mountain meadow of wheel-high wildflowers. I soft-pedaled as my honking and wheezing settled into a heavy pant. When I gathered enough strength to lift my head, I was greeted by a full-screen vision of the Maroon Belles, going off under the luster of the midday sun. I leaned on the trail sign to take it all in. The lactic acid flushed from my legs like Monday morning's coffee down an airport toilet. Hollywood has never written an ending that compares with the summits you come to expect every day on a Lizard Head trip.

BILL STORK

Out of obligation, Tim and John snapped pictures, but fifty mega-pixels or 35mm can only capture the image of a mountaintop in full bloom. The feel of the breeze instantly evaporating the sweat from every pore and the super-saturation of your olfactory by the mountain potpourri are only to be experienced.

This image belongs on the hard drive in your head. It is to be stored in the file with Mom's kitchen, Dad's garage, and reading *The Giving Tree* to your kids.

The wounds and exhaustion inflicted by four hours on the trail are gone like labor pains to a mother cradling her firstborn.

If there are words to describe the triumph of delivering yourself to a mountaintop under hike and pedal power, I'm not the writer to assemble them. The image does not fade.

What goes up, must come down.

"All right men, it is all downhill from here. Literally. We're all tired, we're all beat up. Look to your right, now to your left. We are off the grid. If you go down, it's up to us to get you down. If in doubt, chicken out."

John sensed I was rattled. He clasped my shoulder and headset. "Bro, when you get to the Rock Garden put your chest on the saddle, your butt on the back tire, pick a line, and trust your bike. You've done it before." His focus was penetrating.

He was spot on. Twelve years old and undersized, my Specialized Epic bucked over the boulders like a pissed-off rodeo bull, but I managed to stay on top. Sunshine in the meadow and the scent of agriculture signaled physical safety, though cows don't make the distinction between path and pasture. Tim so accurately called the last mile a shit show. Fenders were more than a suggestion.

The first sensation upon arriving back in camp intact is that of elation, followed very quickly by starvation. In the time it takes to assess my scuffs, cross my chest and give a silent thanks, guides have rolled out a cornucopia of recovery. Bricks of cheese, rolls of sausage, fruits, nuts, and John's turbo-powered guacamole are vaporized in minutes. Dehydrated muscles begging for analgesia and

Vitamin-C pull Orange Peel infused India Pale Ale imported from the Tyranena Brewing Company from their stainless steel camp mugs. Huddled under a tarp and backs to the fire, Mark and the Robs found Rocky's Revenge and the Special Chocolate from the little shop in town a soothing pairing.

Guests retire to their Therma-rests for a late-afternoon siesta. Guides do not so much as break stride. Two bags of Kingsford smolder on a grate. An untreated addict of old school country and bluegrass, I pondered my truck sitting twenty feet away, factory-equipped with 176 stations of satellite radio and concert sound. This moment begged for no digitally downloaded or live-streamed soundtrack. I sat reading Michael Perry's *Jesus Cow*, pausing to absorb the roar of the creek, rustle of the breeze, and the cadence of the cleaver on the cutting board. The sweet-hot and spicy aroma climbed upwind and through my nostrils as the onions and peppers sautéed.

The white-hot coals heated a pyramid of Dutch ovens like Wolfgang Puck's Viking range. In ninety minutes, the cast-iron kitchen bakes a week of road kill veggies, Italian sausage, and lasagna noodles into a delicacy to leave twelve mountain bikers around a campfire bloated and speechless.

There is no humidity at 9,200 feet of elevation to hold warmth. On a cloudless night, when the setting sun perches atop Mt. Crested Butte, bes' put a good quarter chunk of split oak on the fire and go for your Carhartts and stockin' hat.

Cave Man TV: one channel, no commercials.

Four chunks of oak smuggled from the Dairyland and tended by Phil and his scepter throw just enough light so that faces are reduced to broken shadows. The halo of heat binds fourteen folks like a Hindu wedding. Seven are old friends, three are brand new. Family for six days. There are no tweets or posts, only thoughts that have been digested and contemplated. In a voice as deep and smooth as hundred-dollar single malt, Mark the Whisperer dispenses his daily perspective in three sentences or less. I may not remember his words forever, but I will never forget how they made me feel.

If your image of a mountain guide is that of an uber-fit, under-bathed, poorly groomed vagrant, surrounded like Pig Pen by a cloud of pheromones... you're accurate, but incomplete.

What you do not learn until you're making small talk on a hike-a-bike, or gazing across a meadow on a re-group is that their on-the-trail education is underpinned by college degrees in everything from engineering to education, geology, business, and snow science. They're opposed to roofs, walls, and fluorescent lights. They are driven by a passion to share the outdoors with sixty-hour-a-week lowlanders and get us to throw our smart phones to the bottom of a dry bag. Usually at the expense of health insurance, 401ks, and a mailing address.

Their offices are the mountains of Colorado, the deserts of Utah, and the Hill Country of Texas. When he is not riding sweep, loving old yellow labs or managing Lizard Head World Headquarters, Travis guides glacier expeditions in Alaska. I challenge you to find a man in his early thirties who has delivered more Kodachrome moments. He walked away from a full-time gig with 3M to do it. Home is a meticulously arranged utility trailer in Ophir, Colorado.

"What do you call a guide with no girlfriend/boyfriend?"

"Homeless."

Indeed, the lifestyle does not lend itself well to white picket fences and 2.5 kids. When they do pair off and procreate, they raise their children to be more comfortable with a fishing rod or a ski pole than an iPad. Rather than McDonald's Playland or Chuck E. Cheese, they hike, bike, fish, climb and ski.

Joel Paterson has been crowned "the best guitar player in the city of Chicago." If he were to apply his virtuosity to a pipe wrench rather than a Les Paul, he could drive a Lexus SUV to his house in the 'burbs. He drives a ten-year-old Honda Accord and lives in an efficiency.

If Ed Wollin or Ritchie Behm were to take their work day, skill set, and tenacity to town, they could work forty hours and retire with a pension. Yet they must farm.

The same could be said of our friends who guide.

When they are on the road, they work sixteen-hour days. If they are not meticulously coiffed, it is because they are crafting four-course meals, catering to the carnies, vegans and the gluten-free. Their kitchen is two folding tables and a Coleman Pro off the back of a twelve-foot utility trailer, under an easy-up in the driving rain. Once we're fed and paralyzed, they're rebuilding someone's bike under a headlamp with frozen fingers, or scrubbing a cast-iron pot with steel wool.

Meanwhile, Leslie kneads cramped and painful muscles in her massage grotto.

So, it is true that when a guide's lips are in motion, the absolute truth could be at a premium. Trust that s/he's surveyed your equipment, the calluses in your handshake, your profession, experience, and your attention span. Your guide is responsible for fixing your bike if it breaks, and stabilization and evacuation if you do.

Majestic mountain views are a bonus. To push past previously perceived mental and physical limits is defining, contagious, and transcends the seat of a mountain bike.

Marijuana is legal in Colorado. I can think of nowhere that needs less to be enhanced.

BILL STORK

Road Kill

Guidespeak is a language all its own, You will find no college courses; it's only spoken on the trail. One of my favorite terms is Roadkill: the leftover food, beer and provisions that guests leave behind. Often, it's what they live on. In my case, Roadkill refers to the thoughts that wouldn't fit in the flow of the previous story ("You can't handle the truth").

One of the greatest beauties in life is being able to share a place and experience with someone you love. I longed to take Sheila to Camp 4 Coffee, and the Last Steep. I knew she'd love sunset over the Maroon Belles and the wildflowers at their peak. Were it anyone but her, sharing the mountains could have been a problem. Accommodations are primitive, and every moment is not comfortable or dry. She is far more comfortable in the saddle on a Quarter horse rather than pedaling a fully suspended mountain bike.

I warned her of mountain monsoons, smelly bike riders and the outright lack of showers, but her biggest reservation was Remmi. Our thirteen year old lab had been on her last lap for a year, or so we thought. The decision was made in realizing that if our last day was gazing at the Alpine sunset over a mountain meadow, our lives would be complete. We took a bag full of medicine and a cooler large enough for 3 1/6th barrels of Tyranena's finest to the mountains, and (if needed) to bring a sixty pound dog home to the farm.

With anyone else on the planet I would have stressed if her pillow wasn't fluffed. With Sheila committed to go, she'd own the outcome. Still, after two straight days of full-on monsoons, I was a bit concerned.

She claims not to be a bike rider. The upper and lower loop trails are within clear view of Crested Butte, they are still at 9,000 feet above sea level, and have some rather burly terrain. She owned 'em. She rented a mount from Fantasy Ranch, knowing full well it would be more like a merry-go-round with a view, but she never complained. When we saw three cowboys working horses in a corral, she had me pull over. In a phone call and a message she found a seventy year old Italian cowboy with a five year old Paint that she rode into the Black Canyon.

If it is true, "No man stands so tall as when he stoops to help an old yellow lab," then Travis Tucker is 8-foot-4. The day before her thirteenth birthday, Remmi couldn't get up on her own. Rather than bring the group down, we spoke not a word. We were convinced it was her time.

She had tagged Travis as an easy mark the minute she fixed her brown eyes on him, and took up permanent residence under his cutting board. Every time she struggled, he'd scoop her up, steady her, and send her on her way.

John has long professed the healing power of mountain water. Not knowing if we were celebrating her birthday or a living memorial, we drove Remmi up Kebler Pass to Lake Irwin. We were thinking we'd have to carry her to the water and cradle her on shore. She chased a stick and paddled for an hour. Lake Irwin must be a thousand acres of holy water; Remmi chased four tennis balls the next day.

Sheila has no problem getting dirty, but prefers a half hour and a warm shower at the end of the day. I warned her the two options are a solar shower on the side of the van, or melting snow.

A cold shower is the universal sign of a romantic shutout. Immersing oneself on the downstream side of a log damn across Brush Creek, allowing the rushing thirty eight degree water to scrub away a day's worth of excreted toxins is nothing short of a full-on resurrection.

Like two kids dragging their feet into the first day of kindergarten, we snapped pictures of Brush Creek Ranch, a half mile into our journey back to reality.

BILL STORK

"I went a day-and-a-half without knowing where my phone was," Sheila mused as she rolled up the window.

There's no app for that.

Rocky VII

"And there's nothing short a' dying, that's half as lonesome as the sound, of the sleeping city sidewalk..."

I sat close enough to Kristofferson to count the crow's feet in his temples as he winced to retrieve the next verse first written on a bar napkin fifty years ago, or for the pain. The cracked leather of his boots belied the weather in his throaty off-key whisper. A founding father of the Holy Trinity of songwriters, he is known for his poetry and patriotism rather than perfect pitch.

"...and Sunday morning coming down." I was relieved as I looked down the row, my own emotion validated as Scott bent the index finger of his right hand to squeegee a tear down his cheek.

Five thirty Monday morning, the sun will be peeking through the box elder fence line on the east end of Schultz's alfalfa field, like a kid through the railing on Christmas morning. The luckiest herd of Herefords in Jefferson County will be sleeping, swooshing flies, ruminating and fertilizing five acres of fourth crop stubble.

Minutes before dawn, and hours before rain that's not been seen in two weeks, the concentric golden rays diffract the valley fog that hangs in Mud Lake Marsh. The first sign of human life will be Marilyn Trieloff. If there's a flicker of light and a leaf on her lawn, she'll be urgently scampering, in her three-quarter-length windbreaker tied at the waist, picking it up. Just past the first of September, three strands of Christmas lights, a jack-o'-lantern and "Happy Halloween" flicker through the curtains in her living room window.

I'll block the rising sun with my palm, roll down the passenger side and mute Eddie Arnold singing *Cattle Call* on Sirius to study High-

BILL STORK

way 89 South, then turn to my left to give a muted morning wave at Tom Mitchell. He'll mouth "Mornin' Doc" through the windshield and motion me on so he can make the wide turn out of Vita Plus onto 89, headed to Fall River with the first load of feed for the day, or the last of the night.

Casey at a fast trot, and Mojo a slow gallop, will be frantically trying to stay ahead of Laurie Otto taking two sidewalk sections per stride. Their morning constitutional is but a warm-up in her life which makes a cross-fit routine seem like a shuffleboard game.

In the absence of an oncoming car, I hug the centerline to avoid the hot-patched potholes, and hope. "We can begin to measure the true value of society when old men plant trees they will never rest in the shade of." In a year and a half the road will be re-paved. I pray every day we can manage to make room for two lanes, parking, and bicycles without cutting down the trees.

Unless in pursuit of a dystocia, or a down cow, if there is an opportunity to route myself down Main Street, I'll take it. If not, I'll make one. I can't say Lake Mills is the hometown I've always dreamed of, but it is the way I've always wanted to feel. It's all about the people, the lake, and the farms, but every time I pass through town I celebrate the oak and maple canopy like God's own hardwood gauntlet.

Demonstrating that some people retire and others re-purpose, the ageless former school principal Boyd Forest will be riding or running his morning commute across the lake to his son's excavating business.

The overhead door of Steve's Car and Truck Service will throw a rectangle of light into the street, and the backup warning "beep beep beep" will echo between the State Farm building and Blue Moon Pizza, as Junior clears the flatbed and wrecker out of the shop. Like a one-man pit crew at Daytona, he'll have the floor swept and the first O-L-F vacuumed and stickered by six.

Kenny Setz will shuffle under the canopy from the Laundromat searching for the *Wisconsin State Journal*. With the right leg of his jeans cinched by a reflective Velcro strap, a military helmet to the top of his glasses, and a pack on his back with a protruding cardboard tube, "The Natural" pedals furiously up the pedestrian side of Main Street with the focus of Gino Bartali delivering identification documents to Jews in WWII.

As I approach downtown, I will slow to search the shadows. Somewhere on the east side of the 100, 200 or 300 block, there'll be an ageless fixture of South Main Street in camo fatigues and an old-school nylon Badger Hockey jacket, walking his dog, Rocky.

April 22, 2002, is a day that will live in infamy. Brett Favre was in the middle of his sixteen-year tenure with the Packers, and Dr. Stork still felt legit paying for a haircut. It was on that day Rocky Kruse burst through our doors like a 14.8-pound, coal-black, quadrupedal Bam-Bam with ADD and a quart of Mountain Dew. Along for the ride were Paul and Wanda Kruse.

At the Lake Mills Veterinary Clinic, we schedule first puppy visits for at least forty minutes, if not a full hour. It is imperative to ensure that families get a proper start in housetraining, socializing, and caring for their new addition. That they are terminally cute, fun to play with, and make us smile all day is a fortunate perk of the profession.

Rocky's first puppy visit was on the two-month anniversary of his birth.

In her assessment, Dr. Leyla Wirth noted, "Been with owners for two weeks, first puppy, no murmurs, arrhythmias, or hernia, and both testes are descended."

A month later, he returned for his booster immunizations and she noted, "Extremely active puppy, recommend regular exercise and extensive socialization." In later visits Dr. Stork would write, "Extremely sweet, insanely energetic." Dr. James loved to collect puppy kisses. "Nice pup, rambunctious."

Our staff's collective behavioral IQ was not quite prepared for Rocky. It was years before our current staff behaviourist, Mittsy Voiles, would migrate from the Land Down Under. In hindsight, Dr. James Herriot and the pioneering behaviorist Dr. Ian Dunbar could

BILL STORK

have devoted their careers solely to the care of Rocky. Like a freight train, Rocky's path was his own and not to be altered.

We were all just *along for the ride.*

"Recommend regular exercise and extensive socialization," said Dr. Wirth.

Unless there was several inches of firm ice on the lake, Rocky could not be kept out of it. Sentry Steve and others have speculated for years that the pyramidal piles of stones on the bottom of Rock Lake are effigy mounds created by Native American civilizations. Alternate and equally credible theories are that they are a product of Rocky's maniacal games of fetching, diving, and retrieving from the Glacial Drumlin bike trail at the railroad trestle. His canines and molars were worn flat to the gums as evidence.

Unlike the Captain and Tennille, Rocky's relationship with muskrats was anything but warm and fuzzy. In 2006, we were evaluating him for a possible ear infection and ensuring that a few war wounds were healing. Paul noted that he was falling behind on walks. On her list of differential diagnoses, Dr. Clark included early onset arthritis. Her notation was to the effect of, "Suspect degenerative joint disease but difficult to assess due to Rocky's active demeanor."

Owing in some part to his life-long mission that cartographers rearrange the topo map of the lake, Rocky was a frequent flier at the clinic. His appointments were always a two-fer: "Ear infection and radiographs; ate a fish head and lead sinkers," or "Ear infection and evaluate woodchuck wounds."

For the first years, Paul hung on for dear life, and then they walked side by side. Nine years and a month after Dr. Clark made the first notation, with a torn ligament and too many fatty tumors to count, Rocky labored across Water Street. While he waited for the old dog to catch his breath, Paul took a sip from his travel mug. I eased the truck next to the curb in front of the Lakers, offered a feeble wave and swallowed hard to fight back the acid rising in my esophogus.

An hour later, Claire relayed the call I had been dreading for years.

I credit/blame Marilyn Claas for my alarm being set for 4:38. It is thanks to Rocky and Paul that I never hit snooze.

It is an accumulation of small pleasures that get us through the greatest of challenges. Raising my hand and nodding at Paul and Rocky was as grounding and gratifying as a wave from Vernon Strasburg baling hay.

Monday morning, for the first time in thirteen years, they won't be there.

With all due respect to Mr. Kristofferson, there is something half as lonely as a Sunday morning coming down.

The Oxford Comma (and other pertinent affairs of the heart)

Throughout history *journalists* like Edgar R. Murrow, and in my time Walter Cronkite, were cultural icons. I had very little understanding of what was going on, but would not sit down to supper until Mr. Cronkite had summarized the chaos in Vietnam and signed off the CBS evening news "...and that's the way it is."

When he gave his final sign-off in 1981, I was sixteen. The void is as deep and wide as the final episode of *Charlie's Angels*. I expect neither will ever be filled.

Some might say it is skill, *or a lack thereof.* I prefer to believe it is the full-time practice of veterinary medicine, baling hay, and a stout sense of small-town community that has kept our journalistic renown confined to Jefferson and eastern Dane Counties, Wisconsin.

So compared to Murrow, Cronkite, and Koppel, I expect only a regionally adjusted measure of despair in announcing: there is a distinct possibility that this *could* be our final installment in the *Lake Mills Leader*, the *Cambridge News*, and the *Deerfield Independent*.

This announcement could be *a bit* premature, but there is a void to be filled. To portend to fill that void begs a bit of moxie. In my defense, any semblance of bravado is evidence-based. The first printing of *In Herriot's Shadow* sold in less than three months; I am choosing to gloss-over the fact that Don Grant, Scott Clewis, and my dad were responsible for nearly half. In addition, I ran into Dr. Clark's father at her wedding. He's read a few stories and "liked them quite a bit, hey."

You may ask, "Why would you quit now?"

Before he was a stay-at-home father charged with the responsibility of delivering the family 2.9-pound Pomeranian to the groomer for his first blueberry facial (which he prays daily will never surface at a service reunion or the Legion), Dennis Griffee was a highly decorated soldier and true American hero. His military future was sealed when he was a young boy. He watched small children surround his father in his uniform at liberation celebrations while growing up in Europe. Patrick Tillman was an all-pro safety for the Arizona Cardinals. After watching the twin towers fall in September 2001, he turned down millions of dollars in the NFL to serve his country as an Army Ranger.

Unlike the men mentioned above, I do not put my life on the line. Therefore, I stand quietly in their shadows. However, I am prepared for treachery.

Much like Griffee and Tillman, I've been: **Called to Duty**.

In a front page article of the *Wall Street Journal* on Friday, October 2nd, Georgia Wells reported that, after personal hygiene, the second most important criterion in assessing a potential mate at online dating sites is proper spelling and grammar.

I choose to believe her article to some extent, because it brings me comfort. Long before Mittsy broke out the electronic red pen and patched up my fifth grade grammar, I had assumed my empty inbox at eHarmony was solely as a result of my hairstyle. After several spirited exchanges about music, family, and bike riding, a trip to the altar seemed inevitable with "Snuggle Bug" from Cottage Grove. Then, I sent a picture.

My spirits were crushed in one sentence. "I was hoping for someone with hair."

According to Ms. Wells, there coulda been more to it.

Subscribers to Match.com and OkCupid are besieged with profiles and responses written in text-talk, fraught with run-on sentences and spelling errors. According to the WSJ survey, 88 percent of women and 75 percent of men find proper sentence structure

BILL STORK

more important than good teeth. We all have our standards, but I became suspicious the grammar police were attempting to make their case by cherry-picking the data. If a man has a set of hands like a stone mason or biceps like Vin Diesel, and if a woman bears any resemblance to Scarlett Johansson in a sundress, then doubly identifying the subject of a sentence or using an improperly possessive preposition is not gonna leave them at home with a bowl of popcorn and Netflix next Saturday night.

As we have come to expect, I digress.

We are not here to dispute the validity of the *Wall Street Journal*. Whether algorithmically assisted or across the counter at the Kwik Trip, when it comes to affairs of the heart, there are countless variables. We assess body fat, bench press, bowling scores, and dentition, but according to Ms. Wells, if we don't know the difference between their, they're, and there, then we could be resigned to the onerous "table for 1" A travesty of epic proportions.

That is where I hope to apply the collective resources of Blue Collar Dollar Publishing. BCD publishing consists of Mittsy and me (contrary to what the IRS may believe). This being one of my more spontaneous wild hairs, she knows nothing of this venture. We can only hope she agrees, because without her we're helpless. As I alluded earlier, I've written well over 100,000 words in the last five years, yet I would be terrified to take a seventh grade grammar test.

On the other hand, if I have a strength, it was eloquently illustrated in the construction vernacular by my dad: "Well son, if you can't dazzle 'em with brilliance, you can baffle 'em with bullshit." ("Creative non-fiction" per Barnes and Noble.)

As one of his 1,500-pound pet Herefords introduced me to the wall of his pole barn, Dave Messmer asked if I was going to be taking time off to write a novel. He had interpreted the previous week's article in the *Lake Mills Leader* as a farewell. I withdrew from his cow, pronouncing her six months bred, and summarized the findings of the *Wall Street Journal* article, and my intent to try to help.

"Once we roll this thing out," I borrowed a term I heard at a business meeting, "I expect the demand to be overwhelming."

He shared my urgency, "Well, good luck man, I know guys who couldn't write their own name but would do more for a perfect stranger without asking than others might for their best friend on bended knee."

It is those very men, Dave, who lend us purpose.

If I could apply the energy spent constructing the stories and images from *In Herriot's Shadow,* and if Mittsy agrees to correct them, then we could ghostwrite profiles. If just one blue-collar, solo Romeo who "just can't quite put the right words together" could find "that special someone" to share a deer stand with, our purpose would be served.

Statement of intent: We are not above employing artistic license, but I'm in no hurry to get my oak trees tee-peed by a disgruntled client. We may embellish to the point that a lonely-hearted client may be motivated to toss the empty Kwik Trip wrappers from his floorboards, iron his shirt, and scrape his Red Wings in order to get lined up with our propaganda. But we will not make a second string high-school quarterback into Tom Brady, or a past president of Rotary knighted by the Queen.

I would ask that you kindly hold your inquiries. We should wait for Mittsy to agree. Then we'll have to practice. You see these women (and men) who are deleting the profiles of our hard-working brethren are doing so based on a letter designation from A+ to an F, after being filtered through a program called *The Grade.*

That's right, there's an app for sorting suitors.

Then again, I reckon they're doin' *us* a favor.

The "Fall Shuffle"

By way of the interweb, any forward-thinking man or woman can look up the crucial contents of an at-home or on-the-road emergency preparedness kit (EPK).

My friend Dave is a self-proclaimed conspiracy theorist. He bought the Cambridge Ace Hardware. One can never be too prepared.

If you are risk aversive, not up for managing an entire store, or otherwise employed, then UW-extension, FEMA, and the American Red Cross all have extremely complete suggestions. The common, if not obvious, items are bottled water, K-Rations for a week or so, a jar of peanut butter, blankets, flashlights, cell phone chargers, rain poncho, hand warmers and a multi-tool such as a Swiss Army Knife or Leatherman. (Why anyone would go anywhere without a Leatherman is a mystery to me.)

There are personal permutations. The Sheila Barnes Kit would include no less than a five-gallon pail of Clorox Wet-Wipes and ten pounds of pretzels. My friend John lives at 8,800 feet of elevation in Ophir, Colorado. Along with the quinoa, couscous, and Gogurt, he packs an avalanche beacon in his sons Ellis' and Marshall's lunches from Halloween to Easter.

For the environmentally conscious, left-leaning, Subaru pilots, a company called Preparewise offers organic, free-range, and gluten-free EPKs. (Yes, really.) With Amazon Prime, they can be ordered in one-click and shipped the next day for only $229.95 (marked down from $269.95). I sense an untapped sponsorship opportunity for NPR.

The Wisconsin variant on the EPK would include fresh batteries for a radio tuned to WTMJ. There is compelling anecdotal evidence that God is a Packer fan, but it's not our nature to be presumptuous. In the unlikely event a tornado, derecho, or a significant shift of the New Madrid Fault should strike at noon on a football Sunday, we do not want to miss Wayne's play-by-play, Larry's color commentary, and "The Dagger" when the green and gold salt away another Bears evisceration.

They are not called emergencies for nothing.

If your address is anywhere between Lake Michigan and the Mississippi, the Cheddar Curtain and Lake Superior, and if you have an Australian shepherd-blue heeler cross, Jack Russell terrorist, border collie, lab, German short-haired pointer, or equivalent, then your kit should also include a quart of 3 percent hydrogen peroxide, two tablespoons dish soap, and a quarter cup of baking soda.

You will someday find yourself a part of The Fall Shuffle.

Raccoons, woodchucks, opossums, and rabbits generally give birth between May and June. Our children take at least eighteen years to leave the nest. Small mammals hang with their parents until fall, then pair off and seek mates and shelter.

This quest for food, territory, and companionship is what wildlife ecologists call "The Fall Shuffle." (My son Calvin says, "C'mon Dad, we're just hangin' out...")

This instinctive ritual to ensure the perpetuation of the species can result in tunnels to fit a twenty-pound dachshund under your barn if your property is host to a family of groundhogs. These indigenous mammals are mobile in the autumn. They are regrettably oblivious to man's intrusion and propensity to pave their pastures, making them a virtual road-kill buffet for red tail hawks and other raptors.

But these are not, perhaps, the most perilous participants in the fall shuffle. According to Jason O'Brien at the Iowa State University Extension, members of the family mephitis are primarily nocturnal. Well, Dr. O'Brien, evidently north of Dubuque, the striped skunk is not opposed to lookin' for lovin' at dawn, and I have a 2014, gently used, three-quarter-ton Ram Diesel for sale as evidence.

BILL STORK

Early in my years of veterinary practice, Marilyn Claas was always my first client in the barn (unless Dean Frey was milking for Vernon Strasburg). If she had a down cow or dystocia, she'd grab the barn phone and call. I like to consider myself generally of the good-natured type. That said, without a bowl of Corn Flakes and Cinnamon Toast Crunch and ten minutes with yesterday's *Wall Street Journal*, I'm more like a bear with a sore butt. So, by July of 1992, I had settled into 4:38 a.m. as the optimum time to rack out. I can be fed, teeth brushed, "nature" answered, and out the door by 5:30. Marilyn sold her cows twenty years ago, but I'm not willing to take that chance.

Monday, October the 19th...

Waiting for my pupils to adjust in the sepia-toned light of the bathroom off the barn wood floor, I smile at the outline of her form curled softly, the covers gathered 'round her neck. Finding her temple, I pull back a few strands of auburn and kiss Sheila goodbye.

Making just enough sound to have been there, I recede. Accelerating my stroll, I reach for the switches and aim for the bright lights of the kitchen. At the door, Token is chomping at the bit, and Remmi wags, resigned to her sister's ritual.

In mid-October, there is frost on the pasture-yard just outside the bedroom window, a quarter inch of ice on the horse tanks, and five thirty a.m. is darker than a coal miner's crack. There's a moment of silence between throaty howls of northwest wind through the half-dressed hundred year oaks. From beneath the leaves drifted against the wilted hostas comes an innocent shuffle. In a mad dash against November's inevitable permafrost, and fueled by hormones like a pimply high school boy, a young striped skunk digs his den and makes his play.

Since the truck is nearly thirty feet away and I'm obligated by my Y chromosome to carry a week's provisions in one trip, I trap my white plastic afternoon coffee mug between my lower canines and upper incisors. The Stanley vacuum-seal stainless morning mug doesn't leak, so it goes in the back pocket of my coveralls with four strands of baler twine, opposite the Littman Cardio-Pro stethoscope. Its acoustics have been enhanced and the bell cemented in place with dried cow manure. The strap of the laptop bag flung over my head leaves one hand for a pile of neatly folded khakis and Polos for the afternoon of dogs and cats, and the right for a Farm and Fleet bag with leftover LD's brisket sandwich and broken corn chips for lunch.

Right on schedule to start my first set of ab crunches and catch *New Day* on CNN at The Lakers Health Club by 5:55, I hook the loop of the bag on my pinky to wrench the knob open. The door flings against the Culligan dispenser, cueing Token to shoot off like a greyhound after the rabbit. Her pads digging for purchase against the driveway, she takes flight over the concrete deer figurine lying peacefully on the retaining wall.

Token has organized the wildlife on this 6.8 acre swamp in western Jefferson County since she was eight months old. Dubbed "Stork Hollow" by Calvin's friend Thomas, the groundhogs are in their holes under the barn, chippies and squirrels in the trees, and the red fox in the culvert under Wolf Road. Token is convinced that Poe's crows stay aloft thanks to her threat on the ground.

A flock of wild turkeys that look like reverse-evolution in action outweigh and outnumber her ten to one. They get a free pass.

It was as certain as property taxes and prostate exams.

It took six years, nearly to the day. In the face of crisis, I find it useful to maintain a moment of calm. A consequence of inevitability. There may have even been a thread of relief, like catching your son with his first Playboy. Whether it is olfactory or psychological, there is a quick cycle of denial: "Is someone roasting hickory nuts or is the barn on fire?" I thought. Then there was acceptance. The unmistakable hot-in-your-nostrils skunk smell singed the hairs like a marsh fire and brought me near to nausea.

Back from her circuit, Token crouched in "loaded" position next to her door in the truck. She was waiting for the sweep of my finger and saddle up. She had a look of proud satisfaction like she'd just corralled a herd of a hundred Texas longhorns all by herself.

It was going to be a minute.

I bought time doing everything else. I loaded Remmi, put the clothes and lunch on the front seat, took the garbage to the curb, started a load of laundry, swept the garage floor... looking for just one more thing before I had to come up with a plan.

The skunk lecture at the University of Illinois had been twenty-five years ago. If there was more to it than "git the heinous stuff off as fast as possible," I was sleeping. I had hot running water and Dawn in the barn, but my mind scrambled for the proportions of peroxide and baking soda. Charter High Speed Internet would take four minutes to boot, then I'd have to chase down the ingredients. It was eleven minutes to the clinic, where we had a raised tub, respirator, gloves, and DE-SKUNK shampoo.

I made a run for it.

I had endured a few jabs down at Steve's Car and Truck Service when they did the first oil change on my truck and found the heated seats and steering wheel. I reached for some cred and rationalized they'd be a blessing in a blizzard after a dystocia in mid-January, with one of Herriot's lazy winds blowing up the nape of my neck.

Pride was out the window on October 19. It was thirty-eight degrees, and we were hugging the curves on Highway A doing seventy-five, hoping Officer Bob was still in bed. Health papers and back issues of *Dairy Vet* magazine swirled around the cab like confetti in a parade, as we had all four windows and the back glass wide open, like a cross-ventilated hog barn. I had the seat heaters set on medium rare. I hoped somehow that Token would stay in the geographic center of the truck, and touch nothing.

We made it to the clinic in just under eight minutes. Luca and Zoe across the street were in full-throat, but we paid them no heed. I stopped the truck in the middle of the parking lot and flung the doors wide. Remmi's teeth chattered, but her look was "just another Monday with my sister."

Hoping to create some tunnel ventilation, I opened the windows in the waiting room, hub, and kennel as wide as they would go, and reached for a stack of sacrificial towels and the bottle of this magic shampoo we were about to field trial. I pulled a pair of OB sleeves to my armpit, like I was replacing a prolapsed uterus, and reinforced them with nitrile exam gloves. Token's look of smug satisfaction had morphed to uncertain and apologetic. She stood like a sawhorse as I rinsed and repeated until the bottle was empty and the water heater ran cold.

We have the most dedicated and purpose-driven staff I've ever known; this could test them. I stripped the bedding from my truck and threw the towels in the rolling garbage bin, then deposited it in the farthest corner of the yard.

Two weeks out, there's only a hint of the incident lingering in the clinic. According to Darwin, the vile substance "renders all that it touches forever useless." I couldn't have eroded the resale value of my truck further if I smoked fifty cent cigars for the next 200,000 miles and stored retained placentas under the seat.

There will be a time I will stop to appreciate this highly evolved little burrowing mammal. Weighing little more than a barn cat, she's developed an organ capable of shooting a witch's brew of sulfur-containing thiols ten to twenty feet, with accuracy. At point-blank it can cause vomiting and temporary blindness, and can fend off bears. It is detectable by the human nose up to a mile, and can linger in the environment for up to two years.

Any chance at the memory fading is lost every time Token runs through wet grass or in the rain. I ponder. These visually gorgeous little mammals made an indelible impression on The Father of Evolution, and predatory omnivores weighing as much as B.J. Raji are no match for the skunk.

What has prevented them from taking over the world faster than Taylor Swift?

Why was Token unfazed?

BILL STORK

The Farmer and Me

Saturday, October 9, 1986, a group of ten engineering nerds and a token ag student collectively known as the Townsend Two-South "Rhinos" gathered *en masse*.

We marched past the Krannert Center for the Performing Arts. As we crossed Goodwin and Mathews, we trended towards the Natural History Building and Harker Hall. After three years at the University of Illinois, we had learned to give Noyes Lab a wide berth in the fall.

In its illustrious eighty-four-year history, Noyes had produced no fewer than ten Nobel Laureates and polyester. A well-intentioned, yet under-informed grounds crew in the sixties had surrounded the granite temple of chemical engineering with a spectacular grove of ginkgo trees. Likely a gesture to a generous alum, the golden beauty of the maidenhair tree has surely kept them around for 3,000 years.

Like many things, their splendor is best appreciated from afar. On a rainy fall night, the odor of fallen fruit from the female ginkgo tree renders the gauntlet between the ancient chemistry lab and the student union less inhabitable than the penalty box at a pubescent boy's hockey game.

Like a university promo video for diversity, our ten-man contingent cut through the south end of the student union and cashed twenty-five dollar checks to get our cover charge, a few beers, and Sunday night pizza. At the corner of Green and Wright, we superstitiously rubbed a shiny copper spot on the robe of the patina green statue of the Alma Madre, each quietly hoping not to be responsible for her sitting down.

We glanced at the marquis and trotted up the thirty flat black stairs, presenting our student IDs and $3.50. The mountainous doorman grunted and marked the top of our hands with a Sharpie, proving we were twenty-one, or had at least borrowed an ID from someone of the same gender and ethnicity.

We backed away from the door and stood stock-still half across the dance floor. On stage, the Rubenesque lead singer of The Earth Mothers was channeling Janis Joplin and *permanently* expanding our definition of sexuality.

She worked every inch of the stage, like the hippie couple crossing the country "from the Kentucky coalmines to the California sun." Her band and the crowd were just along for the ride.

She softened her shoulders as the bass and guitar decrescendoed. After a twelve-bar break, she fell to the floor and rolled on her back, singin' about when Bobby sang the blues.

She held the bar in the palm of her hand, then hit us between the eyes. As the band rose, she leapt to her feet, growling and crying, "Freedom's just another word for nothin' left to lose..."

And so the evening *began.*

The Earth Mothers were the evening's opening act, followed by a Texas swing outfit that ended rehearsals in time to watch re-runs of *M*A*S*H.* When pressed for a band name, they borrowed from Corporal Maxwell Q. Klinger's hometown minor league baseball team, and The Mudhens were born. Kevin DeForrest was the lead-singer by virtue of his instrumental skills, a gut-bucket baritone, and gift of wit. He was as quick and quotable as Yogi, 6'6", an Olympic-class swimmer, and permanently tan. Ricky and Scott laid down a Texas shuffle like surfin', but the University of Illinois women's swim team dancing and swooning in faded Levis and body suits increased their draw faster than an Amway pyramid scheme.

We left the dorm that night fully intending to celebrate our friend named after a pedestrian traffic violation. On his twenty-first birthday, Jay Walker didn't look a day over twelve. From the three-point line, he was the original Baby Faced Assassin.

We succeeded. The next morning all that remained was my aching head and ringing ears. The head was cured with two glasses of orange juice, three chicken Kievs, and a ten-minute nap.

The ringing *has lasted* twenty-nine years, and grown into a full-blown affliction.

The posted capacity of Mabel's is 365. There must have been 364½, every one of us dancing with abandon. The Bruiser Man seared through his Jimmie Vaughn licks dang near note-for-note, and Barb and I invented the midwest swing on the fly.

Headlining the evening was an overeducated and insanely talented group of original roots rockers called Otis and the Elevators.

After a half-hour set change, Jim Bury, "Natural" Jay Rosenstein, Mark "Toupee" Zehr, and Darris Hess took us all on a ride. Feet planted and eyes just a slit, we pumped our fists to the rafters. "Dominate" was a reggae-infused anthem to those bent on hindering our independence.

Jim once told me, "Bill, always leave 'em wantin' just a little bit more." Just when you thought there was nothing left, he kicked off a four-bar guitar intro and a pregnant pause. When the card-carrying disciple of SRV busted out his take on "Mother Goose," the crowd lost what was left of its collective mind. "Mary had a little lamb," Jim whispered, then croaked, "its fleece was black as coal, yeah!" Midway through the guitar solo, he squared up, turned his back to the crowd, threw his pearl top Strat behind his head, and let 'er rip.

Oblivious to bar time, we weren't going home without "One More Song!" I clapped and stomped my Red Wings and the dance floor thundered like a herd of cattle in an empty hay mow.

Answering our call, Jim and Jay pulled together the members of all three bands. Hoping that collectively they could cobble together all five verses, Kevin started it off. Closing his eyes and creasing his bottom lip he surrounded the microphone like a toddler around a Q-tip: "I pulled in to Nazareth, was feeling 'bout half past dead, just lookin' for a place, where I could lay my head..."

Jim knew, "I picked up my bag, and went lookin' for a place to hide..."

After the chorus, Jay took "Go down miss Moses, they ain't nothin' you can say..."

We all sang the chorus, "Take a load off, Annie, take a load for free," and all ten on stage broke down into harmony for "You put the load right on me..."

After two consecutive refrains looking for the elusive fourth verse, "Toupee" Zehr stepped up like a barefoot Kokopelli with a bass guitar: "Crazy Chester followed me, and he caught me in the fog..."

My friend Jennifer Rodriguez once told me "every interaction changes the course of our life."

I'm not sure, but this one damn sure did.

The theory of parallel instances suggests that there is no such thing as a point source. No fewer than twenty-three people had independently produced a version of the incandescent light bulb by the time Edison threw the switch.

Being as it may, Dr. Bill believes two things:

– October 9, 1986, began my infatuation with all that is art and music, well-written songs and finely crafted imagery.

– And, Bill Monroe is the Father of Bluegrass.

The Mudhens would become the soundtrack of my eight years at the University of Illinois.

For our undergraduation, I asked Dad to bring his twenty-one-foot trailer and every extension cord he owned. The Mudhens could be heard twelve blocks away on Green Street. Seven police officers dropped by to say hi, and for years I met people who were drawn like the Pied Piper. Looking to be good neighbors, we went door-to-door making personal invitations. The old lady across the alley had no ears for blues or taste for barbecue. She was either incorrigible or clever as a politician in a cheap suit: after Buzzard and Quirk had mowed her grass, painted fences, and cleaned the gutters, she conceded to midnight. At 12:00 a.m. on the dot, the 'Hens

BILL STORK

were in full-throat and the gravel dance floor full. Dressed in her nightcap and bathrobe, she shined her Maglight in Kevin's eyes, and waved her finger under his nose. They paused like a blown fuse in middle of a song.

"We have a request, and that is to quit!" Deal's a deal.

The music ended; the party did not.

Three months later, we walked into the University of Illinois College of Veterinary Medicine. At approximately 4'8", sporting dark plastic goggles, and a little bit jaundiced, Dr. Mark Simon was a dead ringer for a two-eyed Minion. He greeted the terrified class of 1992: "Students who are tired perform 27 percent poorer on cognitive tests, 32 percent worse on memory tests, and 25 percent worse on physical tests," he read from a "Haavad" research study.

"So, thay-uh-fore," the tenured professor and Cornell graduate offered his solution, "my advice to you ladies and gentlemen, is *don't get tired.*"

A few weeks into our freshman year of vet school, I was scanning the entertainment section of the Thursday *Daily Illini*. There had been team-building and orientation speeches and receptions by the dean, yet my classmates largely staggered into the lecture hall, heads down, solemn and solo. Thinking this was no way to spend four years, I borrowed a sheet of acetate and a marker. When Dr. Simon returned from the mid-lecture break, there was a notice on the screen:

Class meeting:
Alley Cat
Tonight 9:00PM
The Mudhens

Dr. Stork's research study shows: those who dance together, learn together.

Nearing the home stretch of that first year, I asked Arlin, Rand, and Barb what everyone did after finals. After shoving nine months of drug dosages, muscles, tendons, arteries, and veins into our feeble brains, their response of "go home and go to work" *did not cut it.*

When a puppy sits, stays, or poops in the backyard, we give 'em a freeze-dried liver treat, jump up and down and baby talk until the neighbors think we're crazy.

I called Bruiser.

Four hundred dollars and a gig in a large animal surgery lab was all the incentive The Mudhens needed. A pair of cull sows from swine research wrapped in chicken wire, a dozen bags of Kingsford, and six gallons of Little Porgy's barbecue sauce gave birth to a tradition. After a semester of lectures and labs, and a week of cramming, we staggered into the parking lot, bloodshot, under-bathed, and buzzed on cheap coffee and chewing tobacco.

Big Pat and Little Pat were our chief moral officers and anatomy lab instructors. They tended the coals and sold day-of-show tickets faster than wristbands at the county fair. Setting up the repurposed oil tank smokers ten feet from the intake to the air conditioning for the Basic Science Building was the best advertising since "Where's the beef?" By ten a.m., the fat was dripping onto the coals. Secretaries and grad students were salivating like Pavlov and the research dogs were howlin' like Big Momma Thornton.

The Mudhens disbanded before we could finish vet school. Scott went to Seattle to design stuff with "swooshes," and Kevin moved west for inspiration and love. Bruiser loaded Hedley into the cab, his Strats in the bed of his trademark Toyota, and moved to Austin.

For the week of graduation in 1992, we'd planned to rent the community room at Winfield Village, invite the grandparents and roast another poor hog. Which may have been fine for the CPAs, MBAs or the PhDs, but for this DVM it felt like boneless, skinless, chicken breasts in the microwave for Thanksgiving dinner.

I returned from finals on Thursday, May 13, to a message on the machine: "Hey Willie, this is Arlin," who coincidentally was also in Austin. Like a proud papa, he had planned to come up for the graduation of the class he had so meticulously mentored. Bruiser decided to ride up with him. En route he found out Kevin was going to be in town as well.

"Bruiser was wondering if you had a place they could get together for a gig?"

BILL STORK

They hadn't played together for a few years. Kevin and I scrounged up a PA system.

Before I could pull out of the drive, Kevin stuck his skull through the passenger window. "You wouldn't happen to have an old tape in your truck?"

"Sure." I rifled through the glove box and produced a cassette of *Waxin' the Cat* in a cracked case. "Or would you rather wing it?"

He only got stuck once, shrugging and pointing his palms toward the ceiling tile. I mouthed, *"I like guns and butter, I like potatoes too,"* by which time he was back in the groove: *"I like thinkin' I'm a lovin' man, but I don't much care for you."*

Everybody in the room knew the words to Bruiser's anthem to the lonely man:

I got a pain as big as Texas
I had the blues in San-an-tone
I, once, had a girl, who said she'd always love me,
(rimshot and pause)

The Mudhens' swan song would become the ultimate manifestation of art imitating *and* predicting life.

Four years previous they had played for our undergraduation. We drank, danced and partied, then receded into security of academia.

There would be no more professors over our shoulders. Decisions were no longer graded on a bell curve, but in increments of life and death, love and divorce.

Now it looks like I'm back out on my own.

Game on.

Sunday morning, we turned our tassels. Sunday afternoon, I loaded Cooder and my stereo in the Bronco, had one more rack of ribs at Porgy's, and headed north. Three hours and two tolls later I crossed the Cheddar Curtain, renounced my Illinois citizenship, and bid the Land of Lincoln adieu.

I pride myself in largely maintaining a steady demeanor. Early July 2009, a text from my brother Gary Edmunds had me *all* geeked out: "Hey Willy, Mudhens are doing a Nature's Table reunion on Saturday."

A series of thoughts followed: *Whoa, that's a long drive. What if they aren't any good? I really should mow the grass. I was planning to go on a bike ride.*

Sheila gave me the look.

The Nature's Table was about the size of Shaq's shoebox. It was the organic, veggie, liberal-hippie hangout a block from my dorm. I was taking a study break during finals week late one Saturday night. Sitting elbow-to-elbow on metal folding chairs, I got to tapping my toe a bit too hard and unplugged the vocal monitor as "Workman" Wayne Carter unleased his Ray Charles on the Hammond B-3.

Gluten-free has come a way since 1983. Their bread may have been organic and all-natural, but it took a quart of olive oil (extra virgin) to pass safely. I kept a loaf next to the front door in case of intruders.

Musicians, poets, and bohemians couldn't deny the inevitable march of academic progress. In 1994, The Table was the victim of the wrecking ball. In its footprint stands the Chemical and Life Sciences Lab, but the spirit of the Nature's Table lives on in the hearts of those who performed and those who listened. Each year, grizzled Gen-X musicians gather to play and remember.

Struggling to stifle my memories against expectations, Sheila and I made the sojourn. Had she not fallen asleep, I'm sure I could have filled the four hours with Mudhens stories.

A foot taller than Clooney, but having aged just as gracefully, Kevin took the stage. "Don't worry folks, we've got this under control." He eased our fears. "We rehearsed last night," he barked. "Since we had more beer than time, we only practiced the beginning and the end." Smiling hard, the corners of goatee turned up and the years exposed his crow's feet more. "We cannot be held responsible for what happens in the middle."

The boys staggered through the first few songs, but by the time Kevin boasted, *"Lord, I'm the man all the young girls dream about,"* they had fallen together like a four-man breakaway in the Tour de France. The Mudhens had not played as a band since smoking was legal on airplanes or "the pale blue dot," but they had all gotten sixteen years better as musicians. Honorary 'Hen "Hollywood" Bruce Bethel added a touch of class, wailin' away on the alto sax.

Being given a nickname by Kevin was like being anointed with a trail name on the Appalachian. He said it once and it stuck. The permanence I've come to realize was in his ability to encapsulate a man's entire body of work, in one word.

Bruce Rummenie got two.

As "Natural" Jay Rosenstein changed a string, Bruiser stepped up, snugged his fedora, and closed his eyes. He whipped out his Michael Henderson and took the paint off the walls:

"My baby she left me 'cus I wouldn't put my guitar down..."

When the dust on the dance floor settled, Bruiser gave the crowd a First Communion altar boy nod. Like an overgrown baby brother, Kevin pointed his way and waited for the crowd to silence... "The Boss."

After the show I introduced Sheila. "What you been up to, Big?" Kevin asked.*

This was a time when "stayin' out of trouble" and "same old, same old" wouldn't do.

"Working for farmers and trying to raise a couple kids," I answered, "You?"

"Writing songs."

"Kevin, you may think I'm crazy, but I've been working on this parallel for several years..." I got all excited.

If there was anyone who might get it, we were standing eye to eye. "Starting with you and Bruiser twenty-some years ago, I've developed a healthy measure of respect for, and a number of friends who are musicians, painters, potters, and poets. I get to work for farmers nearly every day. I think there are amazing similarities between the two."

At first glance, farmers and artists couldn't be more different.

Most of the farmers watch the sunrise from the backside. They've got ten-grit calluses and handshakes that'll lighten your heels. They work with impact wrenches, breaker bars, and inch-and-a-half sockets. They take a one-ton diesel pickup truck or a quarter horse to work every day. Their offices are hip-roof dairy barns, free stalls, and the cab of a 500-horse John Deere plowing a 120-acre plot.

They can measure a day's work in bushels, tons, acres, and gallons.

I've grown to be self-conscious about the duration of my pontifications, but Kevin was with me hook, line, and sinker.

Artists work hours that are equal, if opposite. They craft images in notebooks, sketchpads, laptops, and in tons of Paoli Clay pressed through a pug mill. They transport on bike, by foot, or Honda CRV, and their offices are spare bedrooms, coffee shops, or efficiency apartments in Chicago.

They write songs that make us dance, cry, or think. Others craft images in oil of loves lost that will leave you stone-cold and silent.

Kevin drew from a pint of pale ale that looked like a shot glass in his right hand. Then he squared up to me.

Any farmer I know could go to town and work concrete, construction, service, or sales. In half as many hours, they could make twice as much money, and retire at sixty with benefits.

They'd rather be castrated with a dull Newberry knife.

The artists are no different. Mark Skudlarek built his studio, *and* his wood-fired kiln. Joel Paterson and Joe Ely once worked construction. Brad Wells taught chemistry, tai chi, kung fu, and trained dogs.

Yet artists must create, often choosing between sticking to their craft and living in abject poverty, or selling their soul to a barely millennial art director stacking desk toys on her head in the hope of keeping a roof over their heads and health insurance.

Guys in a barn largely talk about weather, women, and the Green Bay Packers. To ask "why do you farm?" feels like inviting them to a Scentsy party or sharing hair (singular) care tips. By now I've spent enough man cards with the writing gig; they're used to me.

Joe Spoke sold real estate before he came back to the farm over forty years ago. He came back to the farm for the love of the land, the marriage of rolling green splendor, and productivity.

Erich Wollin had his feet to the fire as a college sophomore. A 110 mph derecho leveled his family farm for the second time in a decade. If he was going to come back to farm, his father Ed would build it back. He chose to work fourteen-hour days, driven by the variety and the freedom, rewarded by the productivity.

For Ryan Haack, the thought of dairy barns sitting empty with a summer breeze blowing through is depressing. He is rewarded by the physical labor and constant challenge. The idea of not farming is enticing, but frightening. A surprising response for a man who runs 26.2 miles without training an inch.

Ned Healy has four reasons to farm: Sarah, Sam, Keagan, and Vincent.

Productivity, freedom, being outdoors, and family were the recurrent buzzwords when guys looked down at their shoes and kicked the gravel. Yet the knee-jerk, bottom line and the last word is always the same:

"It's just in me."

Mark Skudlarek has probably made 10,000 coffee mugs in his career. My daughter sent a picture of her notebooks, computer, and one of his mugs. The caption: "This mug is my trusted study buddy."

When I shared with Mark, he replied, "You just made it a particularly wonderful morning. Thanks for sharing that, Bill, and my best to Paige."

Bruce Johnson loves to see his work displayed in his friend's home.

I asked Joel Paterson what is his finest reward. "I love to start with a concept, and create a perfect recording."

Catcalls and applause are the tailwind, but ask an artist why they are and their answer is concise. "It's who I am."

I'd held these thoughts close. I still haven't shared them with a farmer. Somehow I think it requires less 'splainin' to compare a song-writer to a dairy farmer than vice versa.

I was not prepared for Kevin's response.

"Damn, Big, you just helped close the loop on a song I've been working on."

A few months later, "Farmer and Me" arrived in my inbox. For a listen to Kevin's take on the parallels between an artist and a farmer, log onto drbillstork.com.

We have stayed in touch by way of Facebook. In April, he posted the release of the first full-length CD by his band Some Train Yard. The Kevin DeForrest I knew was the front man and lead personality for The Mudhens. I was primed to the notion that he had some songs in him by one of his early efforts:

Come on over tonight, let me feel your charms,
Come on over tonight, hold me in your arms,
Did you find that little key, I left beneath your door,
Did you find that little key, and know what it was for.

A fine first effort, especially if you knew the subject about whom he sang. Thirty-some years have cropped his curls and peppered his goatee. They have also lent substance to his lyrics, polished his songcraft, and attracted some mighty talented amigos to accompany him.

True objectivity is elusive at best when a friend has recorded something he's proud of. I played Some Train Yard while doing dishes, folding laundry, and driving four hours down I-39 to Decatur, Illinois, and back.

It just keeps getting better.

My journal sat open on the console of my pickup. Eyes on the road and ears on the stereo, I scribbled notes blindly as I drove. Some of the ones I could read were to the effect:

– vocals are not overdone, or anemic, but completely comfortable

– instrumentals are lush

 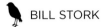 BILL STORK

- what does *ennui* mean?

- he *asked permission* to repeat one of the finest lines I've ever heard

- wow, that's harmony

- that cat can blow the harp

- is that Jerry Douglas on the dobro?

- attention to the breaks, yeah!

- versatility on the mando

- a swing tune on an acoustic album

- all the great hooks *have not* been used

- the biggest influence I can identify on this whole CD is his wife

- DeForrest does not acknowledge the existence of the obvious rhyme or canned metaphor

It was not until four-thirty Saturday morning, sitting on the sun-porch with only the sounds of iron scraping blacktop and backup beeper of the township snowplow to distract me, that I really came to appreciate Some Train Yard.

In a world of digital downloads and live-streamed singles, this is a collection of eleven songs meant to be absorbed from start to finish. Pre-amplified Americana as they are, STY busts right out of the gate with "Old Timey Ennui." An infectious piece that is defiantly upbeat, though the protagonist is anything but happy. Irony runs rampant in the refrain, "I'm as happy as a lark when I hear that banjo bark" and "She's a fiddle playin' baby," though it's Eric Drobny's bass, Bret Billing's dobro, and Kevin Yost's mandolin that move the piece along. Nary a fiddle or banjo to be found.

Song two is an everyman's anthem. DeForrest proves without a doubt that there are still great hooks to be written: "If I'd killed her when I met her, I'd be outta jail by now." No less barroom sing-a-long than "Low Places," but far more gore: "I shot her in the heart, I shot her in the head, I shot her for good measure just to make sure she was dead." This is not to be mistaken for Johnny's Delia. Between Billing's hangman dobro intro and reprise, DeForrest's vocals skip along with Yost's lilting mandolin, making it pretty hard to believe he'd ever go through with it.

Everyone knows to follow up a good murder ballad with a heartfelt profession of love. I've never heard it done more completely than "She's Everything." "She's exactly everything, and everyone, I never knew I always needed." The sentiment is delivered with three-part harmonies and surrounded by Billing's dobro like an overstuffed leather chair.

"Nice to be here" ain't nothin' but a happy song. All by my own self, I was tapping my knee like a high-hat, stomping my boot like a bass drum, and loving the fact the art of a clean break is alive and well. The harp and mandolin feel like a front porch with a screen door where everybody just stops on by.

If you think an acoustic outfit can't swing, think again. Within a few notes of Billings kicking off "Opportunity Knocks," I was doing duck-outs and sweetheart turns with Sheila around the barnwood floor in the middle of a Saturday afternoon.

Don't look now, but Some Train Yard can play the blues. The Jimmy Reed classic "Bright Lights, Big City" is the only cover on the album, and a nice half-time show. I was rockin' rhythm like a train on the tracks right through the harp and dobro call and response, like a man telling his woman, "Go ahead, pretty baby, you don't listen to a word I say."

"If I was the Twilight" is the song Kris Kristofferson would be proud of, Butch Hancock meant when he wrote "Bluebird," and Emmy Lou Harris *must* someday sing. Though the "siren" verse might require a little gender realignment.

A lesser songwriter would be happy to build an entire song around any one of the five metaphors. Like a Kristofferson song, I found myself immersed in an image, only to find he's moved from the shores of the stream to the tracks of a train.

Drobny's three notes down the neck of his bass on the "fiddle and bow" verse sets the tone and speaks to the attention to the song. Yost's mandolin tenderly follows the vocals from verse to verse, and as we've come to expect, Billing's dobro surrounds the whole piece like a mom and her newborn. Just when you think a song can't get any better, we're whisked away by a verse from the gospel classic,

BILL STORK

"I'll Fly Away" dropped in.

"Twilight" is a masterpiece. The song makes me yearn for someone to feel this way about.

"Kickin' Back on The Meramec" made me call my dad and go fishin' for the first time in twenty-five years. 'Nuff said.

There's no better piece for Billing's dobro to drive like a Coupe de Ville on a straightaway, or for DeForrest to do a little growlin', than on the most overtly spiritual song on the album. A dad exposes his own vulnerabilities. "All I know is the Lord likes to work in *Mysterious Ways.*"

"Sadder than Hell" is the lone departure from the overriding positive tone of the album. It is an instrumentally gorgeous piece in which DeForrest laments the commercialization of Nashvegas and the homogenization of country music. There was a day when I would have said, "Damn right, brother!" But I have sat at the feet of a seventy-six-year-old Kris Kristofferson, and at the Bradley Center with 30,000 people listening to Garth Brooks. I've come to realize that just because he's outsold the Beatles doesn't mean he cares any less about "That Summer" than Kevin does about "Twilight" or I do about Fred Eaglesmith's "Summerlea."

Those of us given to coffee shops, microbreweries, listening rooms, and well-thought songs are in real danger of getting a bit righteous. Kenny Chesney came from nothing, loves his fans, and has worked for every dime. If folks get off on "she thinks my tractor's sexy," it can't be wrong.

The hierarchy, bureaucracy, and business of trying to sell a good song is a tragedy.

Some Train Yard sends us home stomping, clapping, and singing along with straight-up bluegrass and the inarguable truth, "If the creek don't rise and we grow old, I'll realize that I've got more than gold."

STY is without a weak link or wasted verse. Not only does it hold up to, but requires repeat listening.

The liner notes are brief: *Each member of the band owns his part and,*

and at the same time, relinquishes that ownership for the greater good of the song.

Yup.

If there's someone on your Christmas list who has hypersensitivity to twang or voluntarily listens to Rascal Flatts, this album is not for them.

If there's someone on your Santa list who gravitates toward song-craft and Americana, Some Train Yard is available at cdbaby.com.

For those of us who born without the fortitude to farm, or the talent to paint, play, or sing... we are eternally grateful.

The farmer feeds our bodies, and sculpts the land.

The artist fuels our soul, and enhances our perception.

*Kevin's "trail name" for me is "Big," though he's a couple inches taller when he stands straight up. My family calls me "little Bill," though I'm several inches taller than most of them.

Live Like You Were Dying

If I should ever lose track of my friend Sheila, I won't have to look in a saloon, salon or strip mall. She's in the barn brushing burdocks, feeding treats, picking stalls or trimming feet. Bennie the two-ton pasture pet and Boom-truck, Stormie, and Big-Butt (Go-Go) the quarter horses are half the herd that currently lives on our seven-acre swamp. Aesculapius has nothing on Sheila Irene Barnes. As she ambles the fifty yards back to our little barnwood berm home, she'll be baby-talking and nuzzling a big gray klutz of a cat named Stinker, while Remmi staggers like "Johnny comes marching home." Meanwhile, Token will secure the perimeter against attack by groundhog, squirrel, or rabbit. Sheila takes a half loaf of Kwik Trip fifty-cent white bread and stale marshmallows up the hill to our ten-year-old Nubian goat named Percy and feeds him by hand.

If I am ever loved half as much as her paint horse Santana or any one of the Wyoming fillies, I will be snug as the Little Nutbrown Hare.

If I ever find myself playing second saxophone to Buckfart, *I'm out.*

Monday mornings, I try to make it to the Lakers "Athletic" (and social) Club by six. The chiseled physique you see is no passive process. I do a half-dozen sets of dumbbell presses and ab crunches while being indoctrinated by the gospel according to Fox Morning News babes, then wander the quarter block south past Blue Moon Pizza and across the alley to Steve's Car and Truck Service and Preachin' Parlor. Forty-five years of fixin', fabricating, towing, and hauling anything that rolls, crawls, or flies have given him forearms like Popeye. A heart like Herriot finds Steve presiding over a small pack of German shorthaired pointers. He collectively refers to them as "assholes," but feeds them hot-buttered whole wheat toast for breakfast. They live in a climate-controlled condo the size of the honeymoon suite at the Holiday Inn, but they are not keen on being left behind. They fight over the dashboard or the bench seat in the Chevrolet passenger van re-purposed from a gymnastics mom.

In the absence of emergencies, by seven-thirty I'm on a thousand-cow dairy owned by Kevin Griswold, where I fear for my *laundry*. In pen one, herdsman Rick's 1,500-pound "girlfriend" number 2308 loves to scratch her poll on the pliers in your back pocket. Rub her right ear or she'll lift you up and dump you in the manure. The Tag Lane Farm's token Brown Swiss lives in pen five. She duck walks like Chuck Berry singing Johnny B. Goode and licks the sky like a golden retriever when you scratch her tail head.

The point of it all being: I work with, work for, and am surrounded by people who love animals... all day, every day.

Given the indisputable notion that folks who are kind to animals are inherently good, that makes Dr. Bill a very fortunate hombre.

Monday afternoon I trade my coveralls for khakis and white lab coat. First up is a rabies shot and stool sample for a lab pup. Tim Esser spent thirty years in law enforcement, yet he was defenseless in his first four months with Trooper. Next door, the tone is muffled like a funeral parlor. Dr. Clark administers a mL of Telazol and last rites, and gives a hug to Wayne, saying goodbye to his eleven-year-old coon dog.

For those who live their lives around their pets, they get to experience the cycle of life several times within their own.

As veterinarians, we participate in that cycle several times a day.

It could be crushing if you let it. It can be beautiful if you choose. It is always impactful.

How much time is left on the clock in our own game of life will dictate just how it affects us.

BILL STORK

When my dog Cooder banked off the rear wheel of the Grand Caravan and could no longer right himself, we let him go peacefully in the whisper grass 'neath the pine trees in the back yard. Paige lay on my back and bawled uncontrollably. For years, she visited his little wooden cross for comfort.

Seven years later, her grandma, with whom she shares her middle name and from whom she inherited her unconditional kindness, was released from the ravages of Alzheimer's dementia. At twelve years old, there was little that could get her out of her hockey pads, let alone into a dark dress and trench coat. She stood like a corner post between her grandpa and me against the granite-gray, stone-cold New Year's Day as the priest crossed himself and we lowered her into the ground.

I knelt before the couch and pressed the bell of my stethoscope against the tiny chest of Petey the twenty-one-year-old Jack Russell terrorist. I held it there long after silence, searching for *other* words. Laura was near eighty years old and had defied the beast that is cancer not once, but twice. She had the strength of 10,000 men and spoke with the voice of reason. "You know, Bill," she paused, "it's tough when you're looking through that same keyhole."

I thought *I* was there for *her*.

In five years and hundreds of thousands of words, I have never hesitated to opine. Yet, I specifically make no attempt to compare the weight of a human life to that of an animal. That said, I find it impossible *not* to apply the experience of knowing, loving, and losing both people and their pets to color and focus the lens through which I view mortality, whether it be my friends, my family, or my own.

Unless I was surgically sterile and elbow-deep in an abdomen, I'd put down my pen or walk away from paying bills when the red F-150 slowed past the office. John Neupert would come around to collect the quarters in the little plastic puppy on the counter for the Jefferson County Humane Society. He always asked about Paige and Calvin, and "How's business going?" His sincerity was well beyond the fact that his bank held the note on both our business and building. I had no clue whether it was his last week, month, or year. John was a family man, lawyer, judge, and Navy pilot. He was a gift to our community; I was proud to know him, and knew he wouldn't be with us forever.

David Letterman asked Warren Zevon how he deals with his diagnosis of lung cancer. He simply responded, "Well Dave, you enjoy every sandwich."

Sometimes there is an acronym. CRF or LSA at the top of your list of pre-existing conditions might motivate a guy to get in his last fishin' trip, motorcycle ride, and "I love you." Bob Sampson was a lawyer who had six kids, served under seven Chicago mayors and presidents Kennedy and Nixon. He wrote much of the Americans with Disabilities Act, was CEO of American Airlines, and was featured with Jerry Lewis thirty-three times on Labor Day weekend. Bob had an acronym on his medical record: MD. He was told he'd never graduate from high school. Not a bad bucket list.

If you are Bill Stork, driving north on Newville Road on the first window-down spring day, listening to Rhonda Vincent sing "Blue Sky Cathedral," you reflect on the decade you were given with The Amazing Dick Bass. If you are Ryan Haack, milking cows off Holzhueter Lane, you lament: if he were still physically here on earth, Brian Jackson just shouldn't be on his mind, every waking moment. He thinks about his pain, and that it is a fraction of what his parents feel. Life will go on; it will not be the same.

It's not supposed to be.

The Amazing Dick Bass and Brian Jackson were taken from us decades before their time. Sometimes the only harbinger is being human: flesh, blood, and finite.

Dispatched to castrate two particularly athletic three-month-old Holstein bull calves, I confessed, "Brian, I don't think I've ever known what you do for a living."

In the process of his explanation, I learned that the eight acres of wooded hillside beyond the calves' paddock was a prairie restoration project. He described that pioneering surveyors like Increase

A. Lapham (yes, the peak) would stand at the stones that marked each quarter-section of land and describe in detail what they saw.

Just short of Thanksgiving, Tim Jeffers presented a particularly delightful German shorthaired cross that he had fostered. Writing health papers takes minutes. As Claire ferreted out the lines I had failed to fill in, we talked Deer Hunting (this is Wisconsin, proper nouns are indeed capitalized), fishing, and faith. The conversation concluded, "Well you know, Doc, it's better to be out on the lake thinking about God, than sittin' in church thinking about fishin'."

Karen Hayes is of stout Norwegian construction. She's had more joints replaced than I've sets of tires on my truck, and been eligible for Social Security since the last Bush was in the Oval Office.

"Good morning. Karen. How are you?" I asked as she stopped for Tri-Heart for Trooper.

"Not worth a dern, Doc." She shook her head. "Getting' old is no fun. Three hours of splittin' wood, and I gotta sit down for a *half hour*." She breaks out in a thunderous laugh and a smile that could clear a cloudy day.

I have no intention of jumping from an airplane or signing up for a rodeo.

What I do try, with varying degrees of success, is to search for, accentuate, and celebrate the beauty within every God-given moment and human interaction. The secondary benefit is if you manage to *not* get hit by a bus, it fends off boredom, and gives a guy great material for a book.

Much like the Monday *New York Times* crossword puzzle, there's the easy stuff. Everybody loves a mid-January hoarfrost sunrise, Ray Charles singing "America the Beautiful," or Scarlett Johansson.

Look for the beauty between. Listen to Glenn Campbell sing Johnny Hartford's "Gentle on My Mind" three times. Pick out Berry Oakley's bass line on The Allman Brothers *Live From the Fillmore East*. Know the smell of freshly plowed ground, and from where the wind blows.

See what you can get done before daylight on December 21st.

My friend Lynn Gustafson was sixteen years old on April 30, 1983, when her neighbor passed away. She had walked over to spend time with his sons when three stretch limousines came to the house. She snuck out the back door, horrified at the sight of a wire-thin Brit climbing out of one of the limos to pay respect. Mick Jagger was followed by Keith Richards, Jimmy Page, and Eric Clapton. Muddy Waters was born to sharecroppers on a plantation in Mississippi, where he learned to play harmonica at age five and guitar by seventeen. He made his way to Chicago. When he plugged his uncle's guitar into an amplifier one Saturday morning so he could be heard above the bartering on Maxwell Street, he set the steel of the bridge between Delta blues and rock and roll. When he returned from touring Europe, he brought with him the British Invasion.

Muddy Waters' funeral proceeded from Maxwell Street to Michigan Avenue. They drank, danced, sang and celebrated his life. Then they laid him in the ground.

At a New Year's Eve gathering, Paul and Dana Ostrowski, Sheila, and I had a cry. In the last weeks we lost Remmi, Jack, and Frida. Earlier in the year we'd said goodbye to Rocky, Brian Jackson, and John Neupert.

Whether it be seventy, thirty-nine, or thirteen, let us not forget the years they were here.

I have never felt the need to form an image of what happens next. Though I don't expect to be met by St. Peter, Dick Bass, and my mom at the Pearly Gates, I do believe that our time on this earth is a part of some continuum. While we are here, we have no idea who we touch, or how.

The steel guitar and fiddles fall silent, and Tim McGraw pauses:

"And he said, Someday I hope you get the chance
To live like you were dyin'..."

I'm thinking maybe today.

Happy New Year.

BILL STORK

A Meditation on Gonadectomy

An extremely predictable confluence of events recently provided me with time to do some involuntary snow-shovel meditation.

Mid-State Equipment in Watertown has custody of my John Deere 2520. Jeff and John are chasing a mechanical version of what vets call a nebulopathy, and I have thirty yards of cobbled blacktop at an 18 percent incline. Which absolutely ensured we would be blessed with the second significant snow event of the season.

The Packers didn't play until 3:15. With a victory over the Maryland Native Americans in the divisional round of the playoffs a foregone conclusion, my mind was clear to contemplate matters of secondary urgency.

I made a double-wide swath down the middle of the drive with the angle-blade and traded for the snow-blaster. As I squatted low and made twenty passes to the west, I pondered how I could benefit society and raise two grounded kids after winning $900 million with my Powerball ticket.

So my fifty-year-old lumbar vertebrae didn't assume a permanent torticollis, I stood upright and slid back to the base of the hill to swipe the other side. With the prevailing northwest wind at my back, I launched snow in the air for Token to attack, and prepared myself on how to answer "the call."

Every author dreams of a book deal from one of the Big Five publishers. After playing to a raucous crowd of eighteen folks at the Lake Mills Public Library (only half of whom are on the payroll), and fifteen minutes on WBEV with Brenda Murphy, I'm expecting one of the next calls to surely be Random House. The conflict is, being a veterinarian takes all my gray matter and most of my time. I love my clients and patients. According to Mike Perry, the life of a best-selling author becomes a perpetual blur of paparazzi, red carpet, readings, and author events. My response time to dystocias, cast-iron furnace grate entrapments, and fish hook entanglements would become too slow to serve. I fear my absence would quickly erode Dr. Clark's chi.

I'm sure the first book deal would be on the same order of magnitude as Aaron Rodgers and J.J. Watt's NFL contracts. In return, the editors at HarperCollins or Simon & Schuster would want to weigh in on the direction and tenor of my little essays. They may have made best sellers and household names of Mike Perry, Bristol Palin, and Mary Higgins Clark, but when I'm looking for a light to follow, I listen to Sylvia Sippel.

For those who follow us regularly (thank you, Don and Gary), our holiday articles reflected on 2015 with a contemplative, and *I thought* uplifting, take on death. The natural sequel would be to wax on the lessons learned in our old dog Remmi's last year, or a re-tread on aging. My son turns eighteen tomorrow.

These notions were shattered with the subtlety of Clay Mathews at a tea party by a woman barely five feet tall and weighing less than the linebacker's equipment.

The door had not shut behind her when Sylvia looked over the top of her glasses. "Live Like You're Dyin', good God man, you gotta lighten up."

Yes, ma'am.

Rather than risk another philosophical, autobiographical tangent, we'll stick to a topic that is both clinically relevant and timely.

It is charming beyond description that many of the young people we know are animal lovers. Rather than iPads and smart rings for Christmas, they begged their parents for puppies and kittens. There could also be a case in which the kids justified mom and dad.

Dr. Clark and I spend the months of January and February ensuring these young 'uns are immunized according to their lifestyle, free of parasites, and skilled at licking our noses. Mittsy, Alli, and

BILL STORK

Danielle teach a puppy class. Graduates of the Lake Mills Puppy Preschool learn that coming to the sound of their name, *not* jumping on people, dropping what's in your mouth, and men in horrifying Halloween masks all result in approximately ten pounds of freeze-dried liver.

The discussion of when *and if* we spay and neuter is a serious one, worthy of tact, clinical facts, and diplomacy. We'll ask, "Have you thought about having him neutered?" Responses vary from "Can you do it now?" to "You can have his if I can have yours."

What follows is a somewhat comprehensive and occasionally serious look at many of the factors we take into consideration as we try hard to make the recommendation that best fits your pet, your family, your relationship with your in-laws, and the dignity of your child's favorite Christmas toy.

Terms used to describe sexual neutralization, in descending order from clinical to the vernacular, include: orchiectomy, spay, neuter, castration, fix, and nut. Others are less elegant. For the purpose of this piece we will use spay and neuter for gender-specific references. Many points will apply equally to males and females.

I'm not a particularly skilled typist, and it seems awkward to reach for the "/" key every time I need to refer to spay/neuter. *Neuter* accurately refers to the procedure in both sexes, but is only two syllables, and evokes less emotion than the British band Coldplay. If Roget says I can use gonadectomy and I choose to use neuter, I'd hope someone would take my laptop next time I get up for a cup of coffee. It takes more time to type, but you can really punch that first syllable. Not to mention, how often do we get to use gonad in appropriate context? My version of Microsoft Word is installed with "redneck spell check," and it still doesn't recognize gonadectomy. It will surely drive Mittsy out of her OCD skull to see so many words underlined in red when I send this to her for editing.

Folks first began to have pets solely for pleasure and companionship in the years after WWII as the nation began to crawl out from under the Great Depression. It surely didn't take long to realize that something had to be done or the country really would go to the dogs. The first and broadest recommendation for neutering was six months of age, largely based on the age at which they were most likely to survive anesthesia. In the few years it took me to get to vet school, anesthesia would become exponentially safer, thanks to pioneering work by the likes of William Tranquilli at the University of Illinois. Still, we stuck with six months, citing studies that demonstrated the incidence of mammary cancer and pregnancies in females spayed before their first estrus was nearly zero.

Those numbers hold up to years and cross-examination, but they are not the only variable to be considered.

Mammary and testicular cancers are prevalent in the population of intact dogs. Gonadectomy at a young age reduces the incidence to nearly zero. There are other cancers such as lymphosarcoma, hemangiosarcoma, and osteosarcoma that may not be recognized by spell check, but are more prevalent in animals that are neutered early as compared to their sexually intact cohorts. It is important to note the actual incidence of these cancers is somewhat breed-dependent, but quite low in general.

Dave Barry would point out that Sexually Intact Cohorts would make a fabulous band name.

We have recently started to look at the effect of early gonadectomy on the incidence of musculoskeletal issues later in life.

Before I began my ascent in the literary world, I considered myself a decent local club bike rider. One fall afternoon, I was furiously pedaling the Glacial Drumlin Trail on my cyclocross bike. As I hunched low, a broken banter through the headwind howled through my helmet (the reader's image of the intensity of the headwind is crucial to my esteem). In short order, I was overtaken like a Prius at Daytona by two pointers and a husky-type dog drawing a repurposed Honda motorcycle frame fashioned in her dad's shop into a three-wheeled chariot.

Reminiscent of Charlton Heston in *The Gladiator,* and at least as attractive, our own Dr. Clark shouted commands like "come by," smiled, and waved as she blew past me.

When there is snow, the same dogs will pull her on skis, sleds, or in moments of minimal organization, her backside. Skijoring and

BILL STORK

sled-dog racing have gotten her a nice collection of medals, some rather stunning bruises (according to Kelly and Kaley), and fueled a keen interest in sports medicine. Dr. Clark is a Certified Canine Rehabilitation Therapist.

Testosterone and estrogen contribute to proper closure of growth plates in long bones of dogs. It is thought that early gonadectomy can increase the likelihood of hip dysplasia and cruciate disease later in life. In guys like Chief, the greatest Dane I know, and Harry the Mastiff, there is nearly universal agreement that delayed gonadectomy is of benefit. As for the carry-on breeds like Pomeranians, Yorkshire terriers, and those microscopic dogs from the Taco Bell commercials who weigh as much as a set of toenail trimmings from their big brothers, we trend toward early neuter.

For the plethora of dogs and breeds who fall in the middle, we work hard to be as inclusive as possible in considering the proper timing of gonadectomy. Owner preference, the dog's personality, conformation, configuration of the family, lifestyle, and fitness are but a few variables we weigh. Your dog's breed is a factor for all the above reasons, as are incidence of certain cancers and diseases.

It's been said there are lies, damn lies, and statistics. The ultimate decision should always revolve around *your dog.*

There are times when the answer is easy and obvious.

Our friends Amy and Ben are the small town Wisconsin, half-scale, 2015 adaptation of *The Brady Bunch*. Because two teenagers, Winston the English shepherd, and eight-year-old Ariel had quickly settled into a harmonious balance, they drove to northern Wisconsin and brought home Henry. At twelve weeks of age, Henry was the golden retriever puppy who truly was cute as a calendar, well on his way to the toilet training hall of fame, and loved to snuggle with his big brother on the front porch.

Regardless of his motivation, it turns out that Henry is as amorous as he is gorgeous. He has taken as his love interest Ariel's stuffed, motion-sensitive, Rudolph the Red-Nosed Reindeer *with* light up nose.

Needless to say, Santa's lead deer takes positive reinforcement light years beyond hotdogs and Velveeta.

Henry will be spending the day with us very soon, and leaving without his two most valued possessions.

There are times when you audible.

Clark Kent and Lois Lane are the couple that give us hope. Shortly after the white picket fence and before the 2.2 kids, they adopted a yellow lab. Bogart had a tail that wagged the whole dog, a head like melon, and charm. Dog's best friend and Mittsy gave the couple advice on establishing proper space with his people. On his second visit it nearly drove him insane, but he knew not to jump up.

But among his buddies at the dog park, his boundaries were still a bit fuzzy. It was determined that a little testosterone might earn him a canine comeuppance. We'd wait to do his surgery near nine months of age.

Factor X, as it turns out, is the in-law's décor.

Jen and John Shipley are Lois' in-laws. They have the most spectacular urban garden, pristine sunset views, a taste for fine microbrews, and a cat that doesn't travel well. I don't so much mind "stopping by on my way home." They've also spent considerable time in New Mexico and Arizona. Their house is warmly decorated in burnt-earth tones, Kokopelli figurines, and Hopi art.

Lois inherited her parent's love of animals, and Bogart was always welcome. Rather, *he was*, right up until he began to lift his leg. His disinvitation was not because the Shipleys were concerned for their carpet. Bogey's first attempted mark was a four-foot saguaro cactus. Weighing sixty-eight pounds at seven months of age, Bogart had grown faster than his vestibular apparatus. Testosterone was telling his brain to mark it a few months before he could reliably balance on three paws.

At the risk of being thought anthropomorphic, I'm thinking the punishment would exceed the crime by a factor of several.

Deere John

Dear John,

This is the letter I *never* thought I'd have to write.

They say, "Nothing *runs* like a Deere,"

It was a John Deere B
With a row crop front end
Hand crank and a flywheel,
The original paint
It won't work another field,
Or farm another farm
Some restaurant up in Omaha's
Got it parked out on its lawn
– Fred J. Eaglesmith from Balin'

Fred could have been singing about the 1935 my Uncle Con used to plant 240 acres of popcorn in Christian County clay and loam, halfway between Stonington and Taylorville, Illinois.

Don Walser sang about workin' a John Deere tractor "ever a day", and Old Shade Tree Slim keepin' her runnin' just fine.

Rest in Peace, Gentleman Don, aka "Pavarotti of the Plains."

My dad started working in Kilborn's John Deere implement dealership his junior year of high school, in 1952. He could have been Ole Shade Tree Slim. He tells stories of fetching tractors from the field and taking them back to the shop for service. There came a call for a '37 John Deere A that didn't sound right. The farmer drove it out of the field, rattlin', back-fartin' and blowing black smoke, onto the single-axle trailer behind a one-ton Chevy dually, with one bolt holding the carburetor, and one holding the cylinder head on the block.

Well there's nothin' like the smell of fresh plowed ground.

There was twice as much fresh plowed ground to be smelling at the end of every day when the 50s and 70s replaced the As and Bs a few years later. With forty-five horsepower at the drawbar, they could handle a four-bottom plow.

After sunset and a couple tablespoons of Talisker, Dad may tell you about going to Lake Shelbyville fishin' with his cousin Jim. Three times. In a row. Show him a picture of an old car, truck, or tractor. He'll tell the make and model *and* that it was made during the first shift, before noon. I'm not prone to challenge his rolling stock recollections, but I swear the first tractor I ever "drove" was a 4020. At five years and fifty pounds, I didn't weigh enough to get on top of the clutch. My legs weren't long enough to straddle the console, so all my toe could reach was the pedal for the inside wheel brake. We lurched, blew black smoke, and headed down the field road. The lugs slow-drummed over hard pack and crunched through gravel as the hundred-horse stalwart rolled with every rut. Leaning on Dad's lap, it felt like I was nine feet in the air, going fifty miles an hour.

Dad swears it was one of Uncle Con's B's (Johnny Poppers) he used to run when he was home on leave from the Navy.

The "put-put" of the Johnny Poppers gets in your blood like the pox virus. When the kids were young, a favorite feature of the early incarnations of Storkfest was a hayride through the backside of Wallace's, all the way to the Muck Farm and back. Dave Strasburg was just on the other side of the alfalfa field and always happy to oblige with an old red or new green tractor, but I figured I'd surprise the old man.

I didn't want to come right out and ask Ed Schulz, so I looked at my boots and kicked the gravel. "Y'all wouldn't have an extra two-cylinder we might borrow for an afternoon?"

The buzz was that he and his son had driven all the way to Canada, and traded a good start at an undergraduate education in American cash dollars for a seventy-five-year-old, fifteen-horse tractor.

They pulled it home behind a Chevy S10 that I wouldn't take to Walgreens for a bottle of Pepto-Bismol.

"Aw, heck, you'd be welcome to it," his John Deere A, *serial number 10*, was hitched to a spreader in a corn crib, "but I got the PTO tore out of it."

It's probably best. Though he is famously collected, the old guy may have lost his mind right then and there. The rumor is the John Deere Pavilion has since offered "significantly" more than what he paid for it. Ed probably thanked 'em for the offer, but he needed it to clean barn.

My neighbor Rich likes to get his two-acre pumpkin patch planted before Memorial Day. My friend Ned rents the ten acres downwind from Applegate Estates, and just across Wolf Road from Stork Hollow.

Michael Perry likens writing to pitching box stalls: "Just keep at it 'til you got a big enough pile someone will notice," says the poet laureate of flannel shirts and work boots. A charming metaphor, but by spring thaw we've got mounds of the real thing.

Though we all may be the same in the eyes of the Lord, all horse shit is not created equally. It gets sorted into three piles.

The hand-sorted pile mixed with pine-shavings that Sheila hauls out in muck buckets I call garden gold. It gets loaded on the trailer and meticulously distributed one wheelbarrow at a time to Jeff and Sharon, Mittsy and Barb, and Nancy and Matt. Sometime after spring showers and the summer solstice, bags of fresh tomatoes, peppers and sweet corn begin to appear on the passenger seat of my truck.

They've got five acres, but Santana and Boom Truck stand just outside the stalls. By spring the fence gets pretty short, and there is a mound of pure manure that gets spread four inches deep on a pumpkin patch across Hwy 18. By Halloween, Rich has jack-o'-lanterns the size of a VW microbus.

The third mound is a nasty mat of wasted hay that gets spread on Ned's corn stubble. Therein lies the fine art and timing of it all: I look for a day with a gentle breeze. Though we are not opposed to wafting a little country potpourri through the cul de sac, they are friends, potential clients, and Dr. Rob from the Jefferson Vet Clinic. A poorly timed gust of prevailing northwest wind as you lift the endgate and you've got Benny's breakfast wedged behind your earlobes, and organic chunks the size of Silly Putty cemented in the mesh of your Packers hat.

Not to mention, I don't need hecklers. Seems every year I find an original and creative way to overload the spreader. At the first smell of burning clutch, I reach for the lever to disengage the PTO. Before turning around to face the inevitable, I'll let fly with a color-ful diatribe that'll surely get me a couple extra Hail Marys and a chuckle from Father Bob, if I ever get back to confession. There will be twenty-five yards of naked stubble and the beaters swinging like Ernest T. Bass with Andy's hand on his forehead. The apron will be stuck to the floor of the spreader, like a flip-flop in stale beer on Sunday morning.

In doing so, I earn an hour and a half's worth of fork-handle-fitness and a bloody blister in my palm. "I can just use the broken-han-dled fork in the jack stand. It'd take too long to walk back to the barn, and all I have to throw off is just that little bit..."

For most, the International vs. John Deere rivalry lies somewhere between Cardinals vs. Cubs and Bears vs. Packers in intensity. On this day, I had six hours before dark, seventeen loads to haul, and Ned was planting corn on Monday. I didn't care if it was red, green, or orange, so long as it had four wheels and a PTO. Sheila's dad usually sends me with the 4020, but the spreader was hooked on the 1937 International M.

I checked the fuel and oil and dropped 'er into road gear. It's eight miles from farm to farm. By way of Highway J to Scheppert Road, you go left onto Perry at the Clampett farm, which will get you all the way to Highway A. By taking Ripley Road, you can avoid the traffic on State Highway 18 *and* get to wave like Huck Finn at the flatlanders opening up their lake cottages, gawking awkwardly as you pull a manure spreader past.

I don't fancy myself all that sensitive. Sheila has gone so far as to say oblivious. I only passed five cars, but three of them had noses

BILL STORK

pressed to the windshield. Another rolled down the window and pointed.

I started to get a little self-conscious.

Once home, I was able to get a notion what the spectacle may have been. I must have been in full-on git-er-done mode. I'm no Scott Clewis, but I fancy myself as fashion forward as a man in the country can be. I was still in Pella Green coveralls and yellow boots from the last farm call, driving a rust red International, while sporting a faded John Deere hat and black shirt. Sheila had forgotten a few things at the farm, so I had her dark brown leather purse, with silver and teal trim, flung over my shoulder.

Folks around Jefferson County, Wisconsin, are cordial toward ag vehicles, though you'll occasionally have a Prius Pete. Apparently, however, when no two pieces of one's ensemble match, folks are far less tolerant of slow-moving vehicles.

When Paige and Calvin were enrolled in the Cambridge School District, I launched a search for a permanent place to hang my coveralls. I hoped for a spot on the bus route, with a little elbow room. Stork Hollow is seven acres of mosquitoes, marsh grass, multiflower rose, and burdock. According to Google Maps, we are at the same elevation as New Orleans.

Sizing up the land restoration project that lay before us, Dad stood on Wolf Road and surveyed the property. "Son, I do believe a guy could walk through there in a brand new pair of Levis, and he'd be buck-nekkid 'fore he got to the other side." Translated: better get some goats.

Aside from a patch of pasture big enough for pickup football or pond hockey, the only flat spot big enough for a pup tent is on the blacktop in front of the garage. After the first snow, the driveway is only slightly less treacherous than the Khumbu Ice Falls.

Paige had begged for a horse since she was five. Aunt Sarah said, "Wait until she's eleven." Just in case, we had four box stalls and a small arena. Her horse fever broke just days before her birthday, but we had plenty of room for four Nubian goats and Bambi the Jersey heifer.

"Family realignment" is a term coined by family practice lawyers. I abhor it, and explained that to my lawyer. We moved my pressboard dressers and secondhand couches from the exclusive St. Vinny's Collection the day after Christmas 2005. Backing the thirty-foot Smith Racing Team car hauler down the bunny hill on solid ice was barely controlled free fall. By the time we unloaded the last box labeled "Blues CD's/Bedroom," the nausea of signing 200 pages obligating me to thirty years at 4.8 percent had not begun to relent. I kept a gallon of kaolin pectin in the truck.

No less prolific or profound, the only thing Mark Twain had on my dad was a measure of eloquence. Though I bet Sam Clemens woulda laid claim any day to, "Son, you can work hard enough to get over stupid; you can't be smart enough to get past lazy."

Dad was not opposed to the classics, "Son, that back of yours has got to last the rest of your life," and "You know, son, you're not getting any younger."

Frugal to a fault, he was no less insistent: "You need to find yourself a little tractor."

Dad had thankfully emerged from his period of P.O.A.D.S. (Pubertal Offspring Associated Dementia Syndrome); I didn't doubt him for a minute. I searched craigslist and the *Tractor Trader* magazine from the wire rack by the diesel pump. As it turns out, good used utility tractors are harder to find than quinoa at a Kwik Trip, and cost twice as much as a signed copy of *Born to Run*.

Worse, they're all orange. The Japanese mastered small-plot farming and have engineered amazing compact tractors to make them efficient. With all due respect, the only Kubotas in Stork Hollow will be borrowed, and as a last resort.

So, until my budget was stronger than my back, snow removal, fence building, and brush clearing would be accomplished by way of a shovel, post-hole digger, and the Stihl Super 028 (*diesel) chainsaw on long-term loan from Dad, fueled by cortisol, testosterone, and bachelor cooking.

Five years after we moved onto Stork Hollow, neighbor Wally saw me dragging brush to the burn pile. Ten minutes later he was out of his business casual khakis and on his twenty five horse Kubota with front end loader. My back was glad for the help, my pride a little dinged.

A year later Sheila showed up with her flaming locks of auburn hair, razor wit, uncommon kindness, *and* a trailer full of quarter horses and a Clydesdale. Dad was *not* willing to bank his chance of scoring a dream DIL on his son's wit, wisdom, and allure.

He made tracks to Sloan Implement in Assumption, Illinois.

Blue collar dollars do not leave my dad's wallet without a hundred hours of hard thought.

I left the University of Illinois with a BS, a DVM, and not a nickel's worth of debt. After Dick Bass and donuts at six a.m., I pitched box stalls and spent happy hours bleaching rat cages for a diminutive Korean named Boon, all of which barely paid for Sunday night pizza and a five-dollar pitcher of Budweiser at Mabel's.

My college education was funded by sweat and sacrifice, and not all mine. Dad worked roughly 6,000 hours of overtime, went on no vacations, and Mom pinched pennies into copper wire. They didn't know new car smell from jasmine tea. The first thing with four wheels Dad ever made payments on was a 2011 John Deere 2520 with a hydraulic bucket, six-foot mower deck, and four-wheel drive. He welded up a four-foot job box that mounted on the draw bar, and painted it JD green to match the rest of the rig.

He hadn't said a word to me.

Word came by way of text from Gary that The Mudhens were having a reunion concert on a Saturday night in Champagne. I called Dad to ask if we could rack at his place after the show.

"Sure. What d'you want for breakfast?" he asked. "Make sure you bring the truck and trailer."

The little diesel ground pounder that now sat in his garage was in hopes of preserving his son's carcass, and a way for an old heavy equipment operator to get his fix.

"When my time comes, I hope they take me mid-stride." The way it's looking, that's the way it'll have to be. When Dad's caught his last crappie, he'll come to rest at the North Fork Cemetery in Decatur, next to Mom. In attendance there will be retired construction workers, machinists, carpenters, farmers, and at least one doctor, lawyer, and Chief Indian.

Long after the eulogy, communion, and Church Lady Food, I'll think of Dad. Every time I clear snow or scrape shit, I'll wing it wide and scrape it tight. Before I start it, I'll check the oil. When the work's done, I'll idle-'er-down, back it in the shed, grease it, scrape the bucket.

It's just the way it's done.

Our John Deere 2520 will be around long after Dad. 'Little Johnny' is his "statue outside the stadium."

The third commandment is, "If *you* break it, *you* pay for it." So, John, there begins what could become a fatal flaw in our relationship.

In medicine, there are what we call nebulopathies. Nebulopathies are illnesses in which the clinical signs are infrequently seen, unpredictable, and can't be reliably reproduced. They may be associated with multiple organ systems and etiologies, but are not directly attributable to a specific pathology. They drive us to spend countless hours cross-referencing cases in the *Journals of Veterinary Medicine* or the Veterinary Information Network, which is occasionally followed by Van Morrison and a two-finger pour of Scotch.

We'll hear, "He was limping all day yesterday, and now he's running around."

Some of our clients are accomplished actors and actresses. They'll bring their hands to their throat, stretch their neck, and emit a guttural hack, then bend at the waist and spread their arms, connoting the phlegm on the floor that terminates the event. It could be kennel cough, heart failure, garbage toxicity, or hairballs.

Mechanics have it tougher.

"I swear the thing goes thucka-thucka-thucka every time I roll down the window," Tom the Roofer tries to describe.

Before he gets around to fixing stuff, Steve always has to grumble,

BILL STORK

"Schuman, you've fallen on your head too many times. Roll up your window and turn up the radio."

We've all had that pickup truck that won't start, dies unpredictably, or loses power when anyone drives it *but* an ASE certified mechanic.

In both veterinary and human medicine we have a distinct advantage: "Put two halves of a sick cat in the same room and they'll get better." The Father of Medicine is Hippocrates. His oath is long, confusing, and written in Greek, but roughly translated it says, "Stay out of the way and we'll get better."

Whether you believe in evolution, creation, or divine intervention, animals are of superior design (the M.S.R.P. of a new Mercedes would lead us to believe otherwise). We can become infected by and exposed to rogue viruses, bacteria, GMOs, and MSG. Just imagine how many times each day we shake hands, share doorknobs, and use public restrooms, and how *relatively* infrequently we get sick.

The defense mechanism of the upper respiratory tract is just one example. It is a system of exquisite design involving fluid dynamics, mechanics, immunoglobulins M and G... and mucus. We can function on only 30 percent of our kidney and 25 percent of our liver function. The redundancy of the circulatory system to the brain is so complete and intricate that we can function perfectly normally with both carotid arteries ligated. Nerves can slowly regenerate and nearly aligned broken bones can heal!

Mechanics have no such luxury.

If it's broken, it'll stay that way until someone replaces the broken parts, sells it, or set it on fire.

One weekend a year we host a down-sized, southern Wisconsin "Woodstock." The horse pasture becomes a parking lot. In anticipation of Storkfest 14, I climbed aboard Little Johnny to scrape a few months' worth of used hay. Our Chicago friend's footwear is more suited for the sideline of a soccer game or the eighteenth green at Medinah; I actually saw a pair of Muck Boots in the tray *next to the front door* of Kish's house. A good tromp through Boomer and Benny's paddock, and I guarantee Anita would relegate them to the garage.

I pulled the bucket-lever back and to my knees to lift and curl... nothing.

Brow creased, I reached for the three-point lever, and slid it back. The collection of T-posts, fencing pliers, and scrap wood in the job box just sat there. Thinking that Little John was one big hydraulic machine, I wiggled the steering wheel and touched the travel, and he did both.

Having an extensive understanding of hydraulics *and* a socket set, I took a drink of the afternoon iced coffee in the cup holder, and dismounted. I rubbed the dust off the little lens next to the PTO to check fluid levels, ran my hand through the sand searching for leaks, and checked couplers and fittings. Finally I remounted, revved the little Japanese diesel to 1800 rpm, and tried the levers again. Nothing.

I have a friend who is a Rolls Royce mechanic. He explained that a Rolls doesn't break down. If ever it should not function, you just make a phone call. I didn't read the fine print, but I suspect John Deere has no such language in the warranty.

Having exhausted my mechanical chops, I dumped down to Plan B: Denial.

After feeding the horses, filling the water tank, and digging the manure away from the posts where the tractor bucket won't fit, I tried again. Success.

Having spent twenty-three years of practice chasing nebulopathies, I was not so delusional as to believe the problem would go away. Old-timers used to take a horse with colic on a therapeutic trailer ride. A couple miles bouncing over a broken down county black-top and he'd let fly with enough methane to power Brookstone Meadows on Super Bowl Sunday, and a pile of manure.

I'd bet a broke-in pair of Red Wings that Johnny could sit there with the bucket on the ground for a week. I'd load it on the trailer and drive to Watertown, and it would work perfectly. They could unplug the quick couplers and drain the hydraulic fluid, and it would still lift a round bale. Load it on the trailer and drive it back home, and it wouldn't pick up a recycled six-pack of Squatters Hop Rising

BILL STORK

Double IPA and an empty milk jug.

I hoped not to be that guy who tries to tell the techs, "Well, this is what it wasn't doing at home."

The service manager at Mid-State was an amiable, if not athletic, slightly aged gentleman named Dennis. He rubbed his brow deeply and repeated the history, "So, Little John starts okay, steers okay, and travels okay?"

"Yes, sir," I said, though my head nodded side-to-side, deliberately leaving silence for thought.

"But the rock shaft and the bucket, he can't get 'em up at all?" he asked without a hint of smirk.

"Sometimes." I shrugged, palms turned toward the ceiling.

It is a well-documented fact that cold things contract. Mechanicals, and especially hydraulics, are famously temperature-dependent.

"Dennis, how about this," I proposed. "In order to ensure he will be symptomatic when we get him to you and Jeff, we wait for a big snowstorm." According to Brian Olson on Channel 15, there was to be a certified Midwestern nor'easter the second week of January. He predicted a foot of snow, temperatures approaching zero, and wind gusts up to thirty mph.

Finally a smile. "Yeah, Bill, that's gotta work."

Snowmaggedon arrived on-time and as promised. I had backed Little John into the garage. If Johnny was feeling good, I could pull straight out of the garage and take the snow between the monument oak and the white picket fence. If not, there was a workout in my immediate future.

I waited patiently for the first four inches to accumulate on the blacktop bunny hill and threw open the garage door. In a click of the ignition, the brief whine of the starter was replaced by an authoritative staccato tenor growl. The smoke curled past the sodium halide yard light and disappeared over the soffit. I pulled my phone from my pocket to check the time. Uncertain what I was praying for and to give Johnny a few minutes to warm and me a few minutes of hope, I lofted the snow from around the garbage cans and recycling bin. Token attacked and eviscerated every shovelful.

I climbed aboard and reached for the bucket lever.

As the onslaught of the storm waited just beyond the garage door, Little John sat, rattling, revving and blowing smoke. I reached for the lever and slowly pulled it to my knee. Like a eunuch at Hedonism during swinger's week… nothing.

Pleased with my prediction but resigned to my fate, I carved a line with my shovel from the garage to Highway 18 and back down. In ninety minutes of Wisconsin cross-training, I had the hill clean, flared wide at the road. In a race against the ongoing storm and the west wind defiantly building a brand-new drift, I backed the trailer and lowered the ramps at the front tires of poor Little John. I had the presence of mind to store the tractor with the bucket six inches in the air. Betting OSHA would not make an impromptu inspection, and anticipating a weather and need-dependent equipment failure (a sentence that a fifty-year-old author must ensure is never cut-and-pasted into his Match.com profile), I could drive right up the ramps.

I left Little John running on the trailer for the ride to Watertown, rather than endure another cold start. I took a lap around Mid-State Equipment and parked next to the "Any equipment left outside of business hours is not the responsibility of Mid-State Equipment, Inc." sign. I positioned the ramps behind the wheels and climbed into the cockpit.

If the Powerball, the stock market, and women were as easy to predict, then Paige and Calvin could have a free ride to the Ivy League college of their choice and I'd be happily married and retire at 62. So predictable was the "Route 26/Interstate 94 Underpass Cure" that my heart rate and blood pressure did not raise a tick, and my diction didn't descend past PG. As soon as I pulled the lever, the bucket rose and curled and the job box hoisted the 200 pounds of split oak I was using for counterweight with ease.

Jeff and Dennis were unfazed. Little John was not the first nebulopathy to cross their shop floor. Their plan was to leave him outside in the cold. Surely, he couldn't get it up, and they could diagnose the issue.

Alas, like a high school boy at a pool party, every time they fired him up, Little John rose to the occasion.

Options were discussed. Little Johnny always works in Watertown. I offered to look for properties north of I-94. But rather than build an ark to relocate five horses, a goat, four cats, Remmi, Token, and Sheila, Dennis offered to engage the expertise of the John Deere technical services team.

Under the direction of "The Green Team," Jeff checked for leaks, performed flow and pressure analysis, radiographs, ultrasound, and blood work. Jeff fed the results of the diagnostics into the computer. According the erectile dysfunction algorithm for John Deere utility tractors, the first differential diagnosis was a faulty tricuspid valve. It would cost the equivalent of open heart surgery, but Johnny was sure to return to full function.

Prepared to relinquish my truck, equity in the clinic, and my son, I approached the cashier. The itemized invoice detailing parts, service, and time looked like the title for Johnny Cash's Cadillac. I winced and turned my head like the little brother in the dodgeball game. "You know Bill, since this is something we've never seen before, I was able to write off *a portion* of the bill as research," Dennis spoke slowly. I opened one eye and relaxed a sphincter. Whether it was generosity or good marketing, I was nevertheless relieved to get out of a John Deere dealership for less than a pair of Super Bowl tickets. I loaded Little John and headed south, grateful and full of hope.

Looking to preserve the feel-good, but still skeptical, I hedged. As long as the weather stayed cold, I stored him in the attached garage and always found something to do for ten minutes while he warmed up. I had no doubt that Jeff had done the best he could. Whether you're a doctor or a mechanic, we try to fix things for good. It's just the nature of the beast.

Little John moved a mountain of manure in the spring, and mowed grass, and augered holes for corner posts all summer. Then came winter. Like a sugar daddy with an expired prescription, by December 2015, Little John was no longer able to get it up.

As a kid, my favorite Saturdays were going to H.H. Donnelly's for parts. Dad was usually rebuilding a carburetor or replacing an exhaust system for the neighbor who had helped pour the concrete driveway or swirl the living room ceiling. Little did I know the smell of wood floors, wheel-bearing grease, and parts cleaner would cement a respect for men and women who 'could,' that would last a lifetime. The chrome stools at the parts shop were polished by overalls and Levis, and the pastel swirls on the Formica counter were worn through by exhaust manifolds wrapped in shop towels. Long before computers, parts were listed in a four foot wide assembly of books and binders on one end of the counter. Dad would always flip me a quarter for the nut hut that dispensed a handful of warm cashews with a turn of the crank.

Old habits don't die. Forty-five years later you can call, email, or text to make an appointment. I'd rather stop by.

Assuming I'm able to stay out of range of Mike Perry's celebrated sneezing cows, Kevin Griswold's Monday morning herd check usually lends just enough organic cred to my coveralls. I don't leave a trail but won't be mistaken for the white-lab-coat-and-khaki DVM.

Not only did I fear the finance, but I also didn't want to disappoint the team who had worked so hard to get Little John back to full function. I was surprised to see a full beard and a young face as the quarterback of the service department. I was daunted at the notion of having to recount the medical history, hopeful that a new set of eyes might be able to resolve the issue.

Evidently, Little John's deficiencies had made it around the break room. Looking at the floor, then the "Payment Expected at the Time of Service" poster hanging above the parts desk, I began, "You may be familiar. I was in last winter with a little 2520…" Like a urologist with excellent bedside manner, John, the young new service manager spoke the words, "Can't get it up, Bill?"

When I hauled Little John the tractor home last time, it seemed we had exhausted the collective expertise of the entire Green Team. I

BILL STORK

was cautiously encouraged by New John's familiarity with my case.

"Bring 'er in, I've got some ideas," he said with confidence. Once out of sight, I raised up on the ball of my foot and skipped half-a-step through the vestibule.

In twenty-four hours he called back with a diagnosis and treatment plan. "Bill, we've taken off the secondary hydraulic pump and found an area that looks as if it got too hot, scarred, and is allowing fluid to back-flow," he said with the confidence of Donald Trump on the campaign stump. "I can't really order parts for the pump. It'd be about $600 for a new one, and the same for the labor to replace it."

"What are our options?" I asked.

"I've got a good lookin' new 270 on the showroom floor, zero down, zero interest, and a full warranty," he said with a smile.

My friend Scott thinks quickly on his feet. He was a high school debate team champion, and has been a very successful lawyer for twenty-five years. By association I learned to withhold the obvious question and build my defense. When I went to pick up Little John, I left my wallet in the truck.

John showed me the offending part. There is a wafer-thin shim the opposing gears seat in, separate from the cast-iron housing. It looked like a glass candle with the flame blown out. "See how it's discolored," he pointed, rearranging his hat.

The service department at Mid-State had worked hard to help; I did not want to make enemies. I said, "From the beginning, the problem Johnny had was that he could travel, he could steer, but he couldn't get it up."

He smiled beneath the bill of his faded green Deere cap and seemed to know exactly where I was going.

"So now, *a year later*, you tell me there is a separate pump for those functions?"

John has soft eyes and an easy manner. He nodded. "Yup."

"*Why was that not the first thing we did?*" I asked with the composure of the clean-up hitter; down by a run, bottom of the ninth, seventh game of the World Series.

His response was as sure as my question. "Because we did what the Green Team told us to do, Bill."

Channeling Scott R. Clewis in a Mayberry RFD vernacular I asked, "John, how many John Deere 2520's do you reckon y'all have in your dealership?"

Getting on board, the office manager called up the file. "A hundred eighty-one," she replied.

"How many *other* machines do you figure have this same part on them?" I continued.

She started to look that up, but it quickly became complicated.

"Too many to count," John agreed.

"Have you ever seen this problem before?" I asked the question for which there was no safe answer.

"Never," he replied definitively.

"You and Jeff have dissected this tractor twice. Is there any evidence it was not maintained properly?"

"Not at all, filters were clean, fluid was clean, fluid was full," he responded.

Knowing a little bit about bypasses and being trained to expect less than your machine is capable of by the best in Operating Engineers Local 965, I continued, "Is there any way I could have used that tractor improperly, and caused the pump part to fail?"

"Not that I can think of," John hedged.

"Well, if Little John has been maintained properly, used gently, and you have never heard of this problem before, then, doesn't this have to be, by definition, a faulty part from the get-go?" I rested my case.

There was a pause. "Yeah," he lifted his cap revealing the beginnings of "crop failure."

I re-acknowledged the tractor was out of warranty. It also had but 221 hours on it, barely a warm up. If it had been maintained and used properly, I needed a plausible explanation as to how it failed before I would have accounting (me) cut the check.

Dennis, John, and Jeff were great. The verdict would come down from above. There would be regional managers and Marvin, in the customer service/warranty department in Moline.

When I sat down to write this piece nearly a month ago, the court of John Deere had not yet ruled. Deere and Company started as a blacksmith's shop in Grand Detour, Illinois. In their second year, they made ten horse-drawn, self-cleaning plows. Last year they produced nearly $40 billion in revenue. I have one twenty-five-horse tractor, two hats, and a T-shirt. I had as much a chance at making an impression on John Deere as the Big Bad Wolf blowing down the Biltmore.

I'm not sure what the original ending was going to be. I'm as likely to Go Red, as becoming a Bears fan.

Last week I got a call from John at Mid-State. "Bill how's about if you pay one-third, we pay one-third, and John Deere pays one-third?"

I reckon you can't get any fairer than that.

He's Baaack...

"This must be the worst part of your job," or "I could never be a vet," owners will say on the dreaded day. There is truth. Not once have I jumped out of bed, and thought, "Boy, I can't wait to go out and put some dogs to sleep today." Equally true is, in the hands of conscientious owners and loving families, euthanasia is a gift. Whether thirteen years or six months, animals who have lived every good day possible do not have to suffer or be in pain until they naturally pass.

It's never easy. And after twenty-four years, there are still tears.

Jenny and Jon Dotzler are the family you hope to have on the other side of the fence. They lived at the mouth of the cul-de-sac, across from the Catholic church, with the requisite two kids and Mikey.

Just as Havoc is the miniature pinscher who doesn't bite, and Brady is the Labrador who won't get wet, Mikey was the beagle who wouldn't bark, bray, or run the other way.

Jenny and Jon are the work-all-week, Saturday morning clients we look forward to. Mikey would stand in the corner of the exam room at the end of a slack leash. At the sound of his name, he'd drum his tail a half-dozen quarter notes between the wall and the hollow-core pocket door. We'd ask about soccer and Little League, while padding the exam table like *The Princess and the Pea*. Mikey knew idle talk. The closer it came to show time, his tail would fall silent. His head would drop fifteen degrees, eyes looking up so all you saw was his sclera, to the extent I apologized to him for every needle.

Mikey had his first seizure when he was four years old. We often don't know the cause of seizure disorders or epilepsy. It can onset

BILL STORK

at any age and can present as subtly as profuse hyper-salivation or momentary loss of awareness (much like conversation with a teenager). Mikey had grand mal seizures, and sometimes in clusters that required late-night runs to the Veterinary Emergency Service. He became unconscious, paddled, and lost control of his bowels and bladder.

Mikey's favorite days were curled up in a chair, sleeping face to the sun, or warming someone's lap. Jenny couldn't feel her feet for an hour after Mikey slept on her legs from Johnson Creek, Wisconsin, to Baltimore, Maryland.

The only drama Mikey ever brought into the Dotzlers' life was completely beyond his control. Unless you consider his love for the peace and splendor of the early morning and his insistence that he share that time with Jenny... and food. Daylight savings or central standard time, made not a lick of difference to Mikey. There was to be a cup of kibble and his small pharmacy of seizure meds in the bottom of his bowl by five a.m., or Jenny was taking paws to the face until the situation was rectified.

Then came Chesney.

If Mikey was a basset hound on Valium disguised as a beagle, Chesney is an ADHD Tasmanian devil on Red Bull... in a beagle's body. But he needed a home, and the Dotzlers are both kind *and* optimistic.

In our first visit, searching for reassurance, I pulled up one of my pearls. (Claire calls them psychobabble B.S. She's helped me recognize when she can do without them.) "You know, one of the inexplicable and beautiful principles of the universe is that animals invariably evolve in the likeness of their families," I said, trying hard to convince myself *and* the Dotzlers. All the while thinking, "Man, I don't even know if Mittsy can help this one."

I have since inserted the Chesney amendment, "Animals *often* evolve in the likeness of their families."

They executed our best advice and took him on leash walks, sometimes from Johnson Creek to Oconomowoc and back. Somehow they avoided the temptation to return with an empty leash. Not a question would be asked or tear shed if Jon had just shrugged, pointed to the vacated collar, and said, "He was there last time I looked."

They took classes and went to dog parks. They gave him Kongs and puzzles to occupy his mind, and Prozac to ease his anxiety. There was hope that by association Chesney might assume some fragment of Mikey's mojo. Instead, he was the little brother who never slept, farted on your head, and punched you as soon as Mom turned around. He would attack Mikey to the point of drawing blood for intersecting his path as he followed his nose around the backyard as he patrolled the perimeter of the fence line. Somewhat understandably, he was especially ruthless when Mikey was still fighting through the fog, after a seizure.

He'd rip toys from Mikey's mouth like the bully on the playground, but when the object of contention was edible, the table turned. Not that the Dotzlers would take any pleasure at his expense, but after dinner when a plate with some residual gravy and a bit of chicken skin was placed on the mat between the two dogs, the kindly Dr. Jekyll would bust out his inner Edward Hyde. Mikey would pin his ears, bare his teeth and back Chesney into Dodge County.

Jenny and Jon are as committed as they are tenacious. At times it seemed they weren't going to sit around and wait for a tumor for "'til death do us part" for Chesney. "Maybe if we just forgot to shut the gate one day..." before their conscience would get the best of them.

When we saw Mikey and Jenny in the evening, it usually wasn't good.

For most dogs, once we are able to establish therapeutic levels of phenobarbital, we see fewer, shorter and less-involved seizures. In Mikey, it seemed that susceptibility to seizure and kindness rode the same chromosome. We increased his dosages and added medications. In the face of all our best efforts, trips to the Veterinary Emergency Service, and intense prayers, the electrical instability in his cute little head eroded his mojo to the point there was no Mikey left.

BILL STORK

On the day Jon carried him into the exam room, Mikey stood on the floor without expression. He didn't look up or down. His head tilted softly to the right and he stared at the baseboard. When we spoke his name, his tail hung flaccid.

The Mikey we all loved had left the building.

I can hold it together when the Carhartt and callused construction guys cry. Still I tried not to look at Jon.

When kids say goodbye to friends they've never known life without, it takes me to the whisper grass under the cedar trees when Cooder could no longer stand. Paige lay on my back with her arms wrapped 'round my neck. With their cheeks pressed together, twelve-year-old Jack Dotzler wrapped his arm around Mikey's chest. I looked through the streaks in the barn dust on my bifocals to find his vein. When I saw the flash, I released the tourniquet and waited between the heaves of the young boy's sobs to push the plunger.

Mikey's chest rose, then his lips fluttered in a final huff. The tears flowed freely as each of the Dotzlers bent to kiss the M on his brow, and tell him, "I love you, Mikey."

The process of mourning is different for every family. We wait for the right one, at the right time. Last Friday, Jenny was on the schedule with a three-year-old terrier cross.

For those of us who ponder the details of *Life After Death,* I present Pepper.

Dear Chesney,

The Bible says, "As ye sow, so shall ye reap."

Dr. Stork says, *sleep with one eye open; your comeuppance has arrived by way of San Antonio, Texas.*

Pepper is 21.7 pounds in a twelve-pound package, all-the-better for ballistics. She's largely white, with a black patch over her eye, easily distinguished from her prey (Chesney). She'd been with the Dotzlers for a year, but I hadn't the pleasure to meet her just yet.

I see Jack Russell terrorist on the schedule and my first thought is "I hope there's a cow with a breeched calf somewhere in the far reaches of Jefferson County, so I can turf him to Dr. Clark's side." My next thoughts are "I'd hate to miss the Dotzlers" and "God would never burden them with Chesney Version 2.0."

I'm glad I didn't try to fake an illness. After meeting Pepper, I'm reworking my tournament brackets. In 128 chances it's never happened, but if a JRT can be as sweet as Pepper, a number sixteen seed can beat a number one. I'm picking UW-Whitewater to beat Kansas in the first game of the South Regional of the NCAA basketball tournament.

Tell Pepper you need blood for a CBC and a chemistry panel and she'll stand like a figurine with her little chin in the air, exposing her jugular vein. Not unusual for a JRT, but for most it's usually a ploy, in order to bring the phlebotomist's nose close enough to rip off. Show her the nail trimmers and she'll present her right paw, flexed at the wrist like Queen Elizabeth meeting Sir Paul. Pull on a glove and lube the index finger and you'll find even Pepper has her limits.

To every respirating, ambulating mammal on planet earth, Pepper is cute as the Pillsbury Doughboy.

Except Chesney.

Two hundred years of breeding fearless little dogs with endless energy in order to bolt badgers, foxes, and groundhogs from their den has been compressed and focused. Pepper wants to play twenty-four hours a day. She'll pounce on Chesney, bite his neck and push off, like Emmitt Smith losing a linebacker. Once she's worn him down, Pepper will sit on a chair, staring at Chesney, daring him to fall asleep. When the first eye falls shut, she doesn't so much as shudder. At precisely the moment the lids touch, she'll go airborne, and latch on just below the collar to ride Chesney around the house or yard. Just when Chesney can't get any madder, she'll disengage.

"You can't hit what you can't see." – Walter Johnson

Chesney'll try to lunge, bite or attack, and all he comes up with is a mouthful of where she hasn't been since yesterday. The poster boy

for learned helplessness, he can often be found curled in his bed...
if Jenny takes Pepper for a walk.

Chesney will soft-walk toward a rawhide, picking the placement
of every paw like a cat stalking a starling. He'll stop short, look all
ways, and rotate his beagle ears. Without so much as an atom of
odor wafting through his olfactory to suggest she's in the area code,
he's all but convinced Pepper has been rehomed. Nevertheless, he's
been programmed not to risk another step. With back feet nearly
off the ground he'll purse his lips to purchase the prize. From nowhere comes a white flash. Left is a blank tile without a trace the
treat was ever there.

Under most circumstances, Jenny and Jon would be on the behavioral hotline to Mittsy for an emergency consult stat.

But, unlike many modern-day incarnations of the Jack Russell terrorist, Pepper is true to the intentions of Reverend John: "An important attribute in this dog was a tempered aggressiveness that would
provide the necessary drive to pursue and bolt the fox (*or Chesney*),
without resulting in physical harm to the quarry and effectively
ending the chase, which was considered unsporting."

For me, there can be only one explanation: Mikey is back, and he's
in the body of a Jack Russell terrier named Pepper.

Reggio "The Hoofer"

Inspired by a vagrant he met in a New Orleans jail, Jerry Jeff Walker wrote the song "Mr. Bojangles" in 1968. There had been a violent shooting in the French Quarter. Police executed a street sweep in order to sort potential suspects. A dancer and entertainer, the man borrowed the moniker Mr. Bojangles from Bill Robinson in order to elude the law. He told of his old dog who "just up and died." I suspect the drunk tank in the New Orleans jail isn't as gay as a night at the county fair. On the request of a cellmate looking to lighten the mood in the room, Mr. Bojangles got up and danced.

Anyone old enough to endure the indignity of a prostate exam can name the tune in one note and hum the chorus. The first cover of "Mr. Bojangles," by the Nitty Gritty Dirt Band, spent weeks in the Billboard Top Ten. It has been interpreted by artists and songwriters from Bob Dylan to Queen Ifrica. Versions have been featured on stage and television by Sammy Davis Jr., Jim Carrey, and Homer Simpson.

The tune written by an intoxicated Texan songwriting poet with a ten-grit tenor has been embellished with orchestras, string sections, and steel guitars behind the angelic voices of Dolly Parton, Emmy Lou Harris, and Whitney Houston.

The song "Mr. Bojangles" couldn't have achieved better market penetration if it had been performed by Taylor Swift holding a puppy rescued from a fire by a former Marine.

I'd bet a broken-in pair of Red Wings that neither Jerry Jeff Walker nor half the generation of folks who can hum the tune knew sickum about Bill Robinson, the original Mr. Bojangles.

BILL STORK

Thanks to a fifty-five-year-old tap dancing ambassador of good will from the south side of Chicago named Reggio McLaughlin, I do.

Bill Robinson was born in 1878. He started dancing and entertaining in the streets of Richmond, Virginia, at five years of age. He was born Luther, but legend has it he didn't care for the name and so he persuaded his brother to trade. His parents died young; Robinson supported himself by dancing, singing, telling jokes and entertaining for anyone who'd throw a nickel at his magical feet. To many, his sixty-year career would parallel the evolution of entertainment in the United States.

In my mind, he helped define it.

He started on church steps and street corners, and made his way from minstrel shows and vaudeville through Broadway, and eventually Hollywood. He is credited for having "brought tap to its toes and making it swing." So much bigger than that, he was also the first black man to: go solo in vaudeville, headline a Broadway show, and take a white dance partner (Shirley Temple). He would become the highest paid African-American entertainer in the first half of the century, but was known by many for his generosity, sometimes subtle. During WWI, he performed gratis for the troops in training camps, and employed Jesse Owens when no one else would. He once paid to have a traffic light erected at a busy intersection in Richmond where he had seen two children chase a ball into the street. He was a fearless advocate for integration and equality. From his platform as a respected entertainer, he petitioned the Dallas Police Department and President Roosevelt for integration and equitable treatment of black police officers and soldiers.

Though skilled with his feet, his heart and generosity would eventually get the best of him. He died without a penny in 1949. Schools in Harlem were closed so children could attend the service. His funeral was arranged and funded by his friend Ed Sullivan; 32,000 were estimated to have paraded past his casket.

Robinson popularized a term. There were shows when the band was tight and the crowd was just right. When the dancers were swingin' and the register ringing, that's when things were "copacetic."

Shortly after his passing, a team of elite dancers was formed to continue the art form and culture of tap. Honi Coles, Charles "Cookie" Cook, and Ernest "Brownie" Brown were The Copasetics. National Tap Day was proposed in 1989. In 2004, President Bush signed into law that May 25th, Bill Robinson's birthday, would be National Tap Day.

At The Old Town School of Folk Music in Chicago, National Tap Day was celebrated on Saturday, June 4, 2016.

Kishan Khemani is a brother; I aspire to his character. Kish is not verbose. Twenty years ago, he arrived at the annual gathering that has come to be known as *Storkfest*.

"Hick, I've got someone I'd like you to meet."

On August 30, 1997, Anita became his wife.

A few years later, Kish called to ask, "Can you be in the city on Thursday, April 17?" He'd already calculated I had to work on the 17th, and it'd take two gallons of coffee and a seven-minute nap to get through the 18th.

The message: just be there.

On that April 17th, I sat at the feet of a songwriting genius. Four grown and accomplished men cried as Kris Kristofferson paused and inflected his way through "Sunday Morning Comin' Down," though we'd heard it a thousand times or more. The cornerstone of the Mount Rushmore of Country Music, *he was opening for* twenty-seven-time Grammy Award-winning Alison Krause, in a room with 325 people.

All that to say, Kish has cred. So, when he picks up his phone to say, "Hick, I've never been so honored to be in the presence of another man in all my fifty years," well, if I portend to tell stories about inspirational people, then I'd better sharpen a pencil, shut my mouth, and get to Chicago.

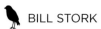

We read about the violence, protests, and politics of Chicago. It is a city of 2.7 million people, bounded by Lake Michigan, the Cheddar Curtain, and The Grain Belt, but it is a collection of communities. Some are defined by economics or ethnicity, and others rise from a shared passion.

One such community is the Old Town School of Folk Music.

To say "Old Town is a school where you can take music and dance lessons" would be akin to "Shakespeare wrote some poems."

Old Town offers lessons from accordion to ukulele, and blues harmonica to beginning contemporary dance. There are classes for anyone from toddlers to baby boomers. Sessions are taught by working musicians, professors, and students of life. A young person at Old Town is in danger of learning skills from finger-picking and proper phrasing to perseverance and respect.

Beginning in 1959, hundreds of artists from every conceivable race, religion, and ethnicity came to a tiny studio in Muscle Shoals, Alabama. Through one of the most racially charged periods in American history, artists ranging from Aretha Franklin to Duane Allman came to Fame Studios. With no regard for race, religion, or orientation, they were there to make music, *together*.

You won't find as many of the names on plaques in Cleveland, but six hundred miles to the north, established 1957, the influence of Old Town School of Folk Music is every bit as significant.

Old Town Director, Bau Graves, handed one of three 2015 Distinguished Teaching Awards to Reginald McLaughlin. Reggio cradled the award like a newborn child. He brushed back his trademark dreadlocks, and let the tears fall to the ground. He thanked his mother for opportunities and the sense to follow them; he credited Old Town... for saving *his* life.

The mentors at Old Town are all masters of their craft. The Distinguished Teaching Award is given to those who help their students master not only andante, allegro, and shuffle ball-change-stamp, but also humility, grace, and gratitude.

I call myself the most underread writer to ever (self) publish a book. If this book were written on the old blue Brother from my high school research papers, I'd need Wite-Out in a fifty-five-gallon drum. With the typing skills of a trained ape and a rather consumptive day job, a healthy percentage of my annual reading takes place during flight delays. "Curling up with a good book" usually results in REM faster than a Monday staff meeting after a midnight calving.

I made it through three of the *7 Habits of Highly Effective People* and *The Purpose Driven Life* is collecting dust. I read *Tap Dance of Life* in two sessions. It's available on Amazon for $19.95. If you don't find a story for the water cooler or your kids, *I'll* buy it from you.

I've always felt there were more people with books in them than those who have written one. Reggio's life story reads more like gospel. After the two-dozenth person suggested, he sat down and wrote *Tap Dance of Life.* An equally appropriate title could have been lifted from Teddy Roosevelt, *Do the Best You Can with What You Got, Where You are, When You're There.*

If you've ever known a veteran of the Depression and World War II, I hope you took time to ask them, "What do you remember?" Wes Gillespie, Bill Dierskmeir, and my grandpa all spoke of family and what they had. Never did they mention what they didn't have. Reggio is one of eight kids, raised by Elsa May McLaughlin, a woman with the strength of 10,000 men and the heart of Mother Teresa.

Reggio walked past a TV when he was seven years old. Mayor Jane Byrne was standing on the steps of what she called "the worst building in the city of Chicago," promising to make changes. He looked out the window to see the television trucks and reporters at his door.

After finishing *Tap Dance of Life,* I sent Kish a text, "I gotta meet Reggio."

The response came two days later. "Be here Saturday at five o'clock."

When he was looking for a home to raise a couple kids, with room for grandparents, Kish had given the Realtor two parameters: within three blocks of Old Town and a baseball field.

We arrived in the last ten minutes of Reggio's Tap 2 class. We sat on the bench outside the classroom as the old building percussed

BILL STORK

on the stomps and rat-a-tat-tat-clap echoed down the hall. From the bowels of the classroom, in a voice like Justin Bieber before his first shave, came, "That was *awesome*, thank you everybody." Old, young, black, white, and Asian, his ten students laughed and tapped their way through the vestibule, wiping sweat like Ali vs Frazier.

Reggio's memory resides in his feet. He can do the Copasetic Soft Shoe, Cane Dance or Chair Dance and read the Gettysburg Address at the same time. Names escape him. He once met the Rolling Stones. By most accounts, their lead singer has a mug that is not easily mistaken. After several attempts, Mr. Jagger resigned himself to being "Nick" for the day.

Off-camber to counter the backpack on his shoulder, he gobbled up floor tiles with a stride I had seen only once before. Michael Jordan also walked as if his feet didn't quite touch the ground, but the purpose in his step was to blow by fans and photographers as if they were a power forward blocking his way to the hole. Reggio's smile stretched between the corn rows that swung like a spastic metronome, and stuck out a hand for everyone who lined his path. "Chief Indian," he growled in recognition of Kish. "Just one second," he excused himself as he walked the length of the hall to thank the janitor and ask, "You doin' okay, man?"

There are words you can't exclude when writing about Reggio; we'll just get them out of the way now: infectious, affable, polite, boundless.

We strode to the Grafton Pub next door where Reggio's entrance was no less grand than his exit from Old Town. Like Norm on *Cheers*, the chants rose from behind the bar, through the swinging doors into the kitchen, and the high-tops in the window, "R-e-g-g-i-o, give us a little shuffle man, don't just walk on by." Reggio worked the crowd from the vestibule to our table. He fist bumped, shook hands and hugged half the people in the bar, asking "How's your mother doin'? Your brother doing okay in school?"

If Reggio's awake, he's on.

We settled into a bench and table. Reggio mounted a chair turned backwards, like a cowboy on a bull named El Diablo. The waiter confirmed, "Mac and cheese, Reggio?"

"You know how I like it, man, thank you *very* much," he responded.

I was hoping for a couple of minutes. Reggio's feet and his heart have taken him all over the world. It was clear that his time was ours. My goal was to ask as few as few questions as possible, wind him up and watch him go.

Not a problem.

On cue, Reggio walked us through a (mostly) seated performance version of his book, *Tap Dance of Life*. As he spoke, I picked cherries. Reggio told of growing up in a building where most boys were shot, stabbed, incarcerated, addicted, or all the above. I asked Reggio how he stayed safe.

"Ah man, you just gotta make friends with the biggest, baddest dude on the playground," he explained. "Not only that, but I had five brothers. You fight me, you fight them."

It was his first installment of "mother wit."

He smiled long enough to stir the steam from his mac and cheese before explaining where he first saw tap.

"Hah," he laughed, "when I got slapped upside the head with a red rubber playground ball." Reggio was seven-going-on-eight when he was distracted from a game of dodgeball at the Chicago School District Recreation Center. He heard a rhythmic shuffle-hop-stamp from behind a partition. He peeked to see a line of girls in shiny shoes tap dancing; he was infected for life.

Reggio taught himself bass when he was thirteen. His brother played guitar, and they enlisted a neighbor boy who had a drum set. They organized a performance in the community room of their building.

At age fifteen he was offered a job as a touring musician.

I knew the answer when I asked, "How hard was it for your mother to let you go on the road?"

"She knew my chances were better on the road with a band than in the neighborhood."

 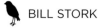 BILL STORK

If opportunities were fastballs down the middle of the plate, Reggio McLaughlin would be hitting .700.

Reggio was learning tap from a Chicago legend named Jimmy Slyde when a friend offered to introduce him to Earnest "Brownie" Brown. Reggio was a student of the history of tap as well as the art. He recognized Brownie as a member of the original Copasetics.

Reggio learned the chair dance and absorbed every subtle step and nuance Brownie had to hand down from Bill Robinson himself. The two were as much a father and son as a dance team. Reggio knows respect. He toured with Brownie until 2009, when Brownie passed.

He was hoofing for tips on the streets when he was hired to perform for a prominent lawyer named Milton Kollman. New York is to tap as Texas is to barbecue. Reggio shared his need to get to the city with Milt. The benevolent lawyer booked him a flight and wrote him a check. As a rough-cut young hoofer from Chicago, they tried to break his spirit. Seeing opportunity where others see adversity, he watched, learned and incorporated everything the hot-shots in the Big Apple had to teach him.

Throughout our dinner, the words blessed, opportunity, and fortunate were in heavy rotation.

Reggio had finished his mac and cheese and second whiskey and Coke, and we had concert tickets.

"Reggio, by my way of thinking, your way out started with that gig in the community room," I asked in the form of a statement.

"Man, I got the first taste of success," he confirmed. "I was not going to let it go."

Thomas Jefferson and ten others are quoted: "I'm a big believer in luck; the harder I work, the more of it I have." That gig and every opportunity in the last forty-three years were a result of Reggio's initiative, attitude, and follow-through.

As we adjourned, I put his feet to the fire. "Reggio, you give credit to your mother, Milt, Slyde, Brownie, and every-damn-body on the planet but Reggio the Hoofer." I had his attention. "You have not seized opportunity, you've *created* it, and you had the good sense to pick the one good choice from a bucket of ten bad ones."

"Ah, Bill, that's just 'mother wit.'" He smiled.

I worked him down to the point he had no choice but to take a little credit for his success. "No man, I appreciate if that's what you think. I ain't gonna go there."

I will.

In college, you listen to your professors, looking to highlight and take notes on what you think will be on the final exam.

In the presence of Reggio the Hoofer, put your pen down and don't miss a word. It's all on the test... called life.

I could not wait to get back home. I sat down to the computer with four pages of scribbles I had made from my time with Reggio. I didn't get a whole paragraph in before I realized there was no way to write about Reggio without actually watching him work.

I mentioned earlier that National Tap Day 2016 was Saturday, June 4th.

Reggio the Hoofer is also a businessman.

My email request to shadow Reggio was returned with a phone call in ten minutes. "So Bill, what's your angle, man? What are you looking to write?"

Suddenly, I knew Reggio left little to chance.

"Where does your writing appear, and how does it get distributed?" He calculated market penetration.

"Well sir, I've got a website, a blog, and appear monthly in several local papers, including *The Lake Mills Leader.*" I specifically attempted not to exaggerate my reach.

I arrived near four p.m. as Reggio had instructed. Dressed in a pair of first generation Air Jordans with laces dangling, and a retro Space Jam baseball jersey falling repeatedly from his shoulders, he instructed me to a seat in the front row before I barely broke the plane of the doorway.

"How you doin' Bill? Good drive down?"

 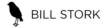

He was in a meeting with the keyboard player. "All right, I'm going to need you to do that intro four times, so I can get my dancers on the stage." And he tapped, working out details one would think may have come up in rehearsal. As it turns out, it was. He beckoned an assistant, "Bring in my tap ones, tap twos and my black shoes."

The dancers and shoes arrived in minutes. The piano man struggled to pick up the beat from Reggio's feet.

Reggio turned to the drummer who had no trouble. Without looking, he instructed, "Y'all sit down and don't ask me questions. I'll let you know when I need you and where."

And he danced.

The band started and stopped on Reggio's cue, and the room filled as he added layers. By now the drummer politely noted even he couldn't hear Reggio's Air Jordans.

Hopping on one foot into his tap shoes, he directed, "Ahh right now, Diane can you get a light and a microphone on the end of the stage for the choir. Don't forget to check levels. I'm going to need some volume on the piano. And where is my man Harrison?"

Where there could be dead air, there was Harrison.

Watching Reggio build the show was akin to assembling a Cadillac by hand while it's rolling down the on-ramp to the Dan Ryan Express Way during rush hour while pulling the parts from a clothes dryer.

I was glued like a gawker's block on the highway, but Kish was coaching his kids' T-ball game a block away. Among the din I gathered my notes.

While directing traffic, Reggio danced his way to the corner of the stage, "Bill, where you going?"

I explained, and he instructed me to be back by six-thirty.

You can search for a new one, but the expression "herding cats" has never been so applicable than watching a White Sox fan, disciple of the discipline of baseball, and consultant to global corporations coach a T-ball game. Though the Tampa Bay Rays hit the ball well, Kish had yet to indoctrinate the kindergartners on "two hands, butt down, and head up." A disparaging word was never heard but the batters up, on deck, and in the hole were helmeted and at attention. Behind the plate, a teenage umpire was calling balls and strikes. I envied him not. I'd rather blow a call against Bobby Knight than muff a T-ball rule against the Chief Indian.

Without anything that resembled a ticket for Reggio's celebration of National Tap Day, I left the game and reported for duty as instructed.

It had been twenty years since Reggio had first proposed that the ukulele player and he should do a show together. The dream came to fruition for the National Tap Day celebration 2016. Then, less than thirty minutes before curtain, it was discovered she could not handle her ukulele arrangement.

As the part was altered on the fly, Reggio the traffic cop pointed to a chair next to the lightboard. "Bill, there's your seat. Enjoy the show."

I already was.

I settled in with my camera and notepad, and the lighting technician stuck out her hand.

"Good evening. My name is Diane. Reggio mentioned you might have some questions."

In sequence, a stately gentleman named Jim offered his hand. Jim is a journalist who helped Reggio assemble *Tap Dance of Life.* He'd be happy to answer any questions I might have.

I thought I was there to watch the people watch Reggio. Alas, if Reggio is in the room, he *is* the show. The production came off without so much as a hitch. Not so much like a fine Swiss timepiece, but more like a Smith family reunion in Pennsylvania. Reggio's productions are not written, rehearsed, reviewed, or revised. From the cast of dancers, singers, and musicians, he builds the foundation on the fly... *then feels it.*

And when there's a gap, he calls on Harrison.

As a fan of old school blues and gut bucket folk music, I've learned people are far more moved by authenticity than virtuosity. You're more likely to put out a canopy fire in a pine forest with a squirt gun than capture a Reggio show with camera and pen. They don't call it percussive dance for nothin'. Next time, I'm renting a seismograph.

Reggio's take on Tap Day 2016 was sensory overload. Master vocalist Sid Brown and the Allen Gressik's Swing Shift Band had but a vague notion what was coming next, but they never missed a beat. From the jaw-dropping athletic art of George Patterson III to ninety-year-old Doris Humphreys, and including every student in Reggio's stable, they brought the house down.

Reggio the Master of Ceremonies executed a half-dozen wardrobe changes and at least as many audibles. From center stage, he commanded the attention of every eye in the crowd and cast.

Harrison took his third encore, and the house lights flooded the room. Reggio's all-encompassing tap family spilled from the auditorium, through the vestibule and onto Lincoln Avenue. I searched and failed to find anyone in the room that Reggio McLaughlin had not touched in a deep and meaningful way, but none more than Harrison.

Four years previous, Harrison asked to participate in his school talent competition. Searching for a skill beyond humming and being silly, his mother showed him a video of *Riverdance.* His older sibs laughed, but Harrison was hooked. His mother approached Old Town, who referred her to Reggio. When Reggio needed to learn tap, he went to New York. When Reggio learned flamenco, he immersed himself in the culture of Spain. When asked to help a special needs boy learn to tap, he jumped in with both feet... and his heart.

I asked Harrison's mother to describe his relationship with Reggio.

"Reggio's determination and love of teaching has been a gift for Harrison." He didn't stop there. Reggio has accompanied Harrison to special needs camps, teaching others the joy of dance and movement.

This was just one night in the life of a man who has danced from street corners in Chicago to Spain and Northern Europe. The magnitude of his impact defies measure.

The Flo-Bert award is given to recognize lifetime achievement in teaching, performing, and supporting the art of tap. Past recipients include Gregory Hines, Gene Kelly, and Savion Glover. The 2013 recipient of the Flo-Bert award is none other than Reggio McLaughlin.

Rest in peace, Mr. Bojangles. Things here in Chicago are indeed Copasetic.

Mother wit is the kind of knowledge that comes from earthly experiences and good old common sense.

Pete

With graduation imminent, Harry Leonard and I sat at Murphy's Irish Pub. Surrounded by profs and students, enveloped in "The Ballad of Curtis Loew" blaring from the jukebox, we were locked in conversation as we had been on surprisingly few occasions in our four years of vet school. Harry is a striking man with shoulders twice as wide as his waist, playful eyes, and a trademark swagger. (I spotted him from fifty yards back at the Western States Veterinary Conference last year in Las Vegas.) He is also succinct. We'd tackle a complex world issue as the bartender pulled a stout, and by the time the foam had settled, it was solved.

I'd conclude, "You know, Harry, life is simple."

After three Guinnesses and several watershed world problems conquered, we parted. So profound were those conversations, it would be a disservice to not write them down. I promised Harry I'd write a book and title it *Harry, Life is Simple.*

In the fall of 2010, I started to write, and in a bout of insanity she surely regrets, Mittsy agreed to edit. We published 300 words a week for the *Lake Mills Leader* and the *Cambridge News*. As of April 2013, I had accumulated fifty or sixty short stories about dogs, cows, and wheelbarrows, birthed from a ragged leatherbound notebook my daughter had given me for Christmas.

If I was going to keep my promise to Dr. Leonard, there needed to be some concrete steps forward. I first stuck my toe into the literary world at The Writer's Institute, sponsored by the University of Wisconsin Continuing Education Department. There were opportunities for agent pitches, publisher pitches, and critique groups. They could have been talking Mandarin. Like going away to a college where you only had one friend from home, I was relieved that Mike Perry was the keynote speaker. I'd figure the rest out.

The session "Book Design from Cover to Cover" seemed about as basic as you can get. Kristin Mitchell and senior designer Dana Gevelinger from Little Creek Press gave an uber-professional yet inviting PowerPoint presentation. They spoke about fonts, formats, ISBN numbers, and proper sizing to fit on bookshelves. Then they passed around children's books like *The Kid Who Climbed the Tarzan Tree* and a lighthearted adult offering, *Blue Jeans in High Places*. Finally Kristin passed a book written by an author named Coleman. *Spoke* is about the civil rights movement in his native Oklahoma. The second I held the book, I knew. I had to publish a book; it had to *feel* like that, in your hand and head.

I approached Kristin after the session like a soccer dad stalking Celine Dion. With my computer bag and notes, I explained that I was working on a collection of short stories by a country vet.

She nodded politely and handed me a card. "That sounds wonderful, Bill. Drop us an email when you get closer."

Mittsy convinced me the venerable veterinarian from England carried a titch more name recognition than Dr. Leonard.

A year later, I sent Kristin the manuscript for *In Herriot's Shadow*. Her acknowledgement explained the book would be sent to one of her editors for approval, or not. A few days later, Kristin forwarded the initial feedback from her editor, who happened to be Coleman himself. There were others, but the comment that stuck was "You must publish this book..."

Game on.

I explained to Kristin that on the first weekend in September, there would be a couple hundred sympathetic friends with discretionary income on my property. It would be crucial to have book in hand by that day. She assured me that would not be a problem.

To follow would be a hundred emails about titles, credits, and a little bird icon to divide the chapters. Kristin and I seem to work similar hours.

As deadline approached, she sent an email. "Bill, I need your 'about the author' for the inside cover by 7:00 a.m.." It was two-thirty in the morning, but I was at the clinic for a tragic euthanasia. She was a bit surprised when I sent it to her an hour later.

Then there was the great cover debate.

Kristin and Dana are masterful graphic artists. It is their work that attracted me to Little Creek in the first place. I explained the feel we wanted for the cover of *In Herriot's Shadow*. Kristin assured me they would produce an image for our book that will be every bit as impactful as *Spoke*.

I had no doubt.

I started to write in order to tell the stories of some of the amazing and inspirational people I've been blessed to know. The process served to elevate my respect for them. I'm often asked in readings about artistic license. My response is "Yes, in order to portray the greatness of my characters, not exaggerate them." More than sales and acclaim, I became deeply motivated to portray characters with the dignity I perceived them.

Glenn Fuller is one such friend: he is my voice of reason and the artist of my last twenty-five years. He was by my side through a hundred Rocky's Revenges at Tyranena, and pretended never to tire as I regaled him with my latest story. He lived *In Herriot's Shadow* from its conception.

Forever humble, Glenn proposed, "So Bill, I'd like to just take some images, massage them a bit, and see what you think. We can send Kristin some *ideas* for the cover."

Roughly translated: *"We got this."*

And so he did. Glenn lurked in the alfalfa field, from the trees, and stood on a ladder around the Haack barn at sunrise, sunset, and high noon.

Meanwhile, Kristin sent images of rolling hills, abandoned barns, sunrises, and sunsets over the spectacular rolling hills near Mineral Point. Every one was a frame worthy piece of art, but not a cow to be seen.

I embraced her reservations to displaying a cover image of a somewhat disheveled barn among the exquisite offerings in her online store, but I dug in like the big guy on the end at a Knights of Columbus tug-o-war.

These are the stories of my people. They're going to be wrapped in a cover that features one of them, rendered by my friend Glenn.

Look closely if you will at the cover of *In Herriot's Shadow*. Past the vestibule of the barn is a man in a blue-green T-shirt. That would be Pete.

Pull down Holzhueter Lane at seven on any given morning, and follow it to its terminus. Look left and you'll find yourself staring into the open doors of the Haack barn. (Regardless of the wind chill, the doors will be wide open. The world in general, and Ryan Haack in particular, lost a friend, Brian Jackson, in the fall of 2015. Brian was not a man whose spirit could be contained within walls and a roof. With the open door, Ryan feels closer, even if it means freezing his fingers.)

I mentioned Pete only briefly in *In Herriot's Shadow*. It was well below zero with crushing windchill on a day I was dispatched to the Haack's to service a cow. On that day, the doors were closed and frozen hard. I bull-hunched them open and fell into the vestibule, dropped my bucket, and pulled them shut. A cosmetic move at best; the cracks in the boards only served to accelerate the prevailing northwest wind.

The first thing I heard was, "Merry Christmas, Doc Bill," as I turned to see a smiling Pete, knee-deep in the gutter, trying to free a frozen barn chain, gray water dripping from his chin.

And so it goes. Total stranger or lifelong friend, if Pete is on the farm, he'll come busting out of the barn and knock on your window. "How can I help, are you lost, tired, hungry, out of gas, flat tire?"

Pete Milburn is the first guy to offer up a hearty, "How you doin', Doc?" He's also the guy who could use one the most.

Pete works(ed) third shift at Oscar Mayer, pressure washing and sanitizing production equipment. There's no need to shower or change clothes when he's done with his ten-hour shift. He staggers to his car, grabs a Mountain Dew, and heads eighteen miles east down Interstate 94. At the Haack farm, he milks cows, cleans, and feeds calves. I've seen Pete run headlong into the front porch of the house, thirty paces north of the calf barn. Pete has sleeping skills my dad can only aspire to. Dad can fall asleep standing up. Pete can do it while walking, with a five-gallon bucket of milk replacer in each hand.

Working back-to-back Mike Rowe jobs could break the spirit of any mortal man or woman; for Pete, it's recreation.

To the put-upon housewives on Oprah and in Ann Landers who lament husbands who don't do their fair share around the house, I present Pete.

The Milburn household has yardwork, laundry, and cleaning, just like every family of four. The difference comes at meal time. For years, Pete's son has battled the effects of a disorder called mito-chondrial storage disease. Especially during onslaughts, his body can't assimilate the nutrients he takes in. As a result, he becomes weak and loses cognitive function. Pete and his wife Kristin have taught him how to walk and read at least three times.

As you might imagine, the impact on a family is enormous. MSD is a genetic disorder that is exacerbated by stress. Five years ago, the symptoms began to manifest in Kristin. So now, Pete feeds both his wife and son through feeding tubes.

Two years ago, Kristin was also diagnosed with malignant mela-noma. Oscar Mayer and the union tried to build a case to have him fired when Pete missed too much work taking Kristin to Cancer Centers of America for treatment. Given a prognosis of weeks to months, Kristin was not supposed to make it to last Christmas. She missed the memo. Social Services informed them their best chance at state aid would be to get divorced because Pete made too much money.

The reason this image *had* to be the front cover of *In Herriot's*

Shadow is that the Wisconsin DOT estimates there are 60,000 vehicles that pass within clear sight of those barn doors on the Milwaukee-Madison corridor every day. I will wager a pretty penny not one knows Pete's story. We can't cure mitochondrial storage disease and can only treat malignant melanoma. Bill Gates' money would not make the pain go away.

What I implore us to do is live in a fashion that is sensitive to the notion that every one of us is carrying a load. It could be physical, mental, emotional, or financial.

Pete knows more hardship on Tuesday than many of us will in a year, but in no way does that diminish our own struggle.

What I'm asking is that we borrow a small piece of Alma Ann Stork, my mom.

Friend or perfect stranger, when she asked *"How are you doing?"* what she really meant was, how can I help?

BILL STORK

About the Author

A veterinarian by trade and a keen observer of the American experience, Dr. Bill Stork has an innate ability to see the best in people and appreciates the simple pleasures of a life well lived.

Stepping from Herriot's Shadow is his second book. His first, *In Herriot's Shadow*, was published in 2014.

In his books, Stork delivers powerful accounts of people, places and things that many others would allow to go unnoticed. His stories are not those of politicians or titans of industry, but rather of ordinary folk who are not so ordinary upon closer inspection.

Stork's father said he never learned a thing with his mouth open. That friendly curiosity has been passed on to the son.

At various points in his life he's answered to Bill, Billy, Bill Bill, Little Bill, Willie, The Hick, Daddy, The Professor, Dr. Bill, Dr. Stork – and still does to this day. This book would not exist without Mittsy Voiles, Glenn Fuller, Robb Grindstaff, and many he's encountered throughout his journeys.

Since writing his first book, Stork has been humbled and honored to meet his readers at local bookstores, pet wellness expos, and winter festivals where he signs and sells books. Each has story of their own to share and Stork is always more than happy to listen.

The author says he's been buoyed and encouraged by critics – some complimentary, some not so much. As a result, his appreciation for those who bank their existence on their artistry and craft has risen exponentially from its already sky high levels.

A 1992 graduate of the University of Illinois College of Veterinary Medicine, Stork currently lives in Cambridge, Wisconsin, and is the owner-operator of the Lake Mills Veterinary Clinic in Lake Mills, Wisconsin.

When not writing or wrangling animals, he can be found engaged in multi-day bicycling tours, tracing the roots of American music through the Deep South, searching for the perfect piece of beef brisket, or simply having a pint at the local brewery.

Like a fine bourbon, his stories are immediately entertaining, but even more enjoyable upon reflection.

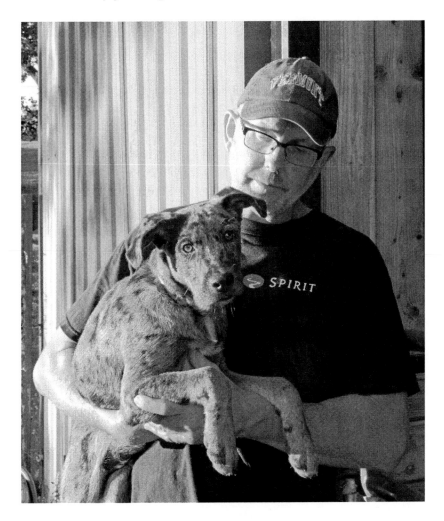

Acknowledgements

I am grateful that folks who favored our freshman effort were first to the party. I always knew there would be someone out there who was not so charmed. In that regard, I would like to thank Sarah W. Keegan for stepping up.

Her criticisms felt like closing my thumb in the car door the first few times I read them, but she made valid points. I even had to look up *tome,* to ensure I surmised the right meaning. This book will have animal stories right out of the gate, thank you Sarah. I am still a person of faith (though challenged recently); I will not back down from that perspective. As for the good old days, I'm going to cherry pick the beauty from every generation as I see it.

Possibly the most meaningful comments on *In Herriot's Shadow* have come from Wayne and Nicole Howie. Wayne is not a frequent reader, as providing for his family and raising three kids takes up most of his energy. Though it took complications from what was supposed to be a minor surgery to put him on the sideline, when he found himself resting with a bag of frozen peas, he read my book. In addition, Nicole read chapters to their children Myles, Adilyne, and Haydn. Adilyne asked why there were no pictures. On Nicole's suggestion, she and Myles busted out the scrap paper and crayons. The best seller list and Pulitzer would sit on the shelf second to those Crayola masterpieces.

Just wondered if there was any special reason I could not find your column in this week's Leader. – Sylvia

Our friend Sylvia is a poet to whom I can only aspire, and capable of brevity that I often choose to avoid.

I first thank Robb, Joyce, Matt, Scott and all the good people at the *Lake Mills Leader, The Cambridge News,* and *Deerfield Independent.* The business of producing a quality local newspaper is a herculean task in the age of all things instant and digital. From the outside, it seems the editors do everything from cut down the trees to delivery. At a reasonable rate they offered me valuable space in their papers to tell my stories and scratch the itch that started with John Boy Walton and James Herriot.

These stories are conceived in the cab of my truck, in the seat of my tractor, and armpit deep in a cow with a breached calf. Thoughts are scribbled on scraps of paper and a half-dozen mangled spiral notebooks from high school and a fancy leather-bound parchment one gifted by my daughter. They are assembled in the roughest of fashion in the hours before the Sunday sunrise. I would be terrified at the notion of an 8th grade grammar test and wouldn't print an editorial in *The Onion* without first being patched up by my editor, Mittsy Voiles. I send her between 1,200 and 3,000 words a week; she picks 380 good ones, and sends them on to the paper.

Kathleen Dunn introduced me on Wisconsin Public Radio as an author and veterinarian. I consider myself a vet blessed with a stable of exemplary friends, perspective, and support. Janet Peterson once told me, "You know Bill, I've driven the same roads and known the same people as you, I never knew what I was missing." Thanks Janet, mission accomplished. I'm more comfortable reserving the *author* title for folks like Mike Perry. The sum of his acquired skills and fortitude puts food on the table and gas in the tank.

There are far more folks with books in them, than those who have written one. When an introduction at a signing or reading begins, "I've always wanted to write a book," I defer. One of our early stories was conceived in a blizzard on Christmas morning and revolved around a farm hand named Robbie.

After "Take Notes Kim Kardashian" appeared in the *Lake Mills Leader* DonMary Grant pulled me aside in the parking lot of the clinic and said, "Doc, I love the humanity in your writing." Mark Twain once said, "I can live two months on a good compliment." *That one* resulted in a book called *In Herriot's Shadow*.

To follow would be John at London Lumber, Dave Messmer, Charlie at the Tyranena Brewing Company, and tens of others. To resonate in the hearts of those you admire and aspire to, is the ultimate validation and motivation to put words on these pages that are worthy of the ten minutes it takes good people to read them.

To anyone who has read, commented, or shared... Thank You.

I'd like to thank Michael Clish at WFAW, Brenda Murphy at WBEV, Orv Graham at WKOW, and Kathleen Dunn at WPR. In the age of digital and free, the business of terrestrial radio is bloody at best. These people took the time to read *In Herriot's Shadow*, asked insightful questions, and allowed me to help build my brand.

On the topic of free and digital, and in the face of Amazon I am grateful for our local brick and mortar bookstores and coffee shops. They are vital businesses on our main streets, give people a place to gather, authors to be featured, and often have great cinnamon rolls. That list includes but is not limited to Mystery to Me, Tribeca Gallery Café & Books, Books and Company, Arcadia, Edgerton Books and Art Store, Waterhouse Foods, Camrock Café, and wherever the hell else I've been.

It is impossible to over-value small town libraries. They are perpetuated by tireless friends groups and are an outlet for self-published authors. Thank you to the library staff of Lake Mills, Jefferson, Fort Atkinson, Palmyra, Marshall, and Johnson Creek.

Thank you to Tyranena Terri, Ilse, Patricia Sampson, and all the other incredible people I've met while peddling the book.

BILL STORK